# SUGGESTION
# OF THE
# DEVIL

JUDITH S. NEAMAN was born in Syracuse, New York, in 1936. She received her B.A. from the University of Michigan in 1958. She attended Columbia University in 1959 and received her M.A. in American literature in 1960, completing her degree with a thesis on the aesthetics of Henry James. After teaching for two years she returned to Columbia to pursue her doctoral studies in English and comparative medieval literature. She received her Ph.D. in 1968.

Throughout her graduate school studies, Dr. Neaman was drawn to Columbia's "history of ideas" approach and found medieval studies particularly appealing because of the necessary synthesis of art, history, science, and literature. Her approach to medieval studies was highly interdisciplinary long before that was fashionable. She has written articles and papers on astronomy and poetry, liturgy and romance, and brain physiology and rhetoric. She has designed graduate interdisciplinary courses, the most enjoyable of which she found her "test course" for this book, "Insanity, Literature and Society in Ancient Greece, Medieval Europe, and Modern America." She has taught at Lehman College, Hofstra University and Hunter College and is the co-author, with Dr. Rhoda Nathan of a critical anthology in American studies, *The American Vision: The Individual and Collective Modes,* published by Scott Foresman in 1973. Maintaining that she must compensate for being the "wrong kind of doctor," Dr. Neaman is now at work on her second book on medieval medicine and society.

# SUGGESTION OF THE DEVIL

## *The Origins of Madness*

Judith S. Neaman

Anchor Books
Anchor Press/Doubleday
Garden City, New York
1975

Library of Congress Cataloging in Publication Data

Neaman, Judith S
  Suggestion of the Devil

  Bibliography: p. 205
  Includes index.
  1. Psychiatry—History. 2. Medicine, Medieval.
3. Insanity. I. Title.
RC438.N4      362.2'09'02
ISBN 0-385-08569-9
Library of Congress Catalog Card Number 73-9041

Anchor Books Edition
Copyright © 1975 by Judith Neaman
Printed in the United States of America
First Edition

*To Peter and Adam*

# NOTE

This book is addressed to an audience which includes both specialists and general readers. The psychiatrist, psychologist, medievalist or social historian who wishes to pursue the topic further will find the sources of my materials in the chapter notes at the end of the book. The notes are not essential to the text itself and anyone who wishes to do so can read the text without interruption or consultation of the notes.

# ACKNOWLEDGMENTS

This book grew out of some graduate research, completed in 1967 and supervised by Professor W. T. H. Jackson of Columbia University. To Professor Jackson and Professor Howard Schless, a second adviser, I am grateful for assistance and patience long ago, with an only semi-literary topic ahead of its day. Subsequent research was immeasurably advanced by some postdoctoral studies in canon law, supported by a grant from the National Endowment for the Humanities, and I am thankful for their faith and funds in times of research poverty. I also owe a debt of gratitude to the rare-book librarians, especially Mrs. Alice Weaver, of the New York Academy of Medicine, who were always helpful.

Mr. Solomon Smith of the Yale Law Library and Professors Thomas Waldman and Edward Peters, both of the University of Pennsylvania, were generous with time and suggestions. Mrs. Marion Cavoli was diligent, inquiring and endlessly scrupulous in her intelligent translation of the major portion of the canon law quotations. Barbara Hohol, who typed the manuscript rapidly and efficiently, was also most accommodating throughout.

Last, among my lengthier acknowledgments, I am happy to count four people without whose encouragement and aid this book would never have been possible. Elizabeth Knappman is a remarkable editor with vision and independence. Her faith in this project and her incisive professional skill were a constant inspiration to "do well" and "do better," as Piers Plowman wished. Professor Carol Silver was a creative listener and an understanding friend. Her editorial advice and comments were both essential and ingenious. Finally, my husband, Peter, and son, Adam, the first who was always a true believer, encouraging and helpful in innumerable ways, the second who learned to understand my work and his own importance with the simultaneity of a remarkable person, merit an epic dedication.

My general thanks are due to friends and colleagues who were both resourceful and concerned: Ellen Lynn, Hannah Alexandra Achtenberg, Dr. Rhoda Nathan, Barbara Graber, Dr. Ellen Robinson, the Drs. Wagman, Dr. Arthur Root.

# CONTENTS

# SUGGESTION
# OF THE
# DEVIL

# INTRODUCTION

Each of the three declared he was Christ and predicted the coming of the end of the world. Each had been sent to earth to teach and knew that he, as Christ, must suffer martyrdom. Fearing their presumptions and violent convictions, their three families placed them in the care of those who might treat them kindly. These guardians provided living quarters for them—a small mattress, a bare room, a cement floor, a dim light. Doctors listened to them, inquired about their fears and hopes, and tried to expose the unreality of their beliefs. But the three Christs clung to their private visions.[1]

Their visions were more apocalyptic than those of a young medical student who became equally obsessed. One day the student left his studies for a swim in a nearby stream. Emerging from the water, he found his body covered with leeches. Overcome with terror, he plucked them off but remained convinced he had swallowed one leech. Before he reached his room, he was talking wildly to himself. His fellow students watched his fear lapse into depression. His teachers recommended him to therapy. The therapists reasoned with him, eliciting his confession of terror. Their attempts to calm his fears were useless. Finally, one therapist suggested he have the leech removed by surgery. After the student was put to sleep, the surgeon removed a dead leech from a jar and placed it on the pillow beside him. When he awoke he found the leech, and was convinced it had been removed from his throat. He was restored to mental health.

When did each of these incidents of insanity occur? The three Christs are modern Americans who were treated at the Ypsilanti State Hospital for the insane. The medical student acquired and lost his obsession in the twelfth century. Medieval madmen were not all confined in dank towers: it was the twelfth-century student who was treated in his normal environment while the twentieth-century Christs were condemned to cheerless gray cells.

Cheerful pragmatism, ingenious solutions and a willingness to meet the patient on his own terms are not the exclusive domain of the enlightened twentieth century; it was the medieval doctor who, temporarily entering into the reality of his patient's perceptions, arrived at a rapid and clever solution to the problem. The three Christs were condemned to a world of denial because they were unreasonable. Yet the three Christs and the twelfth-century student all belong to the community of the mad. In their paranoia and their delusions, which we call psychosis, they bridge all centuries. Their delusions are ours and so are their fears. Their delusions are those of power and victimization and their fears are of death and doomsday.

Psychotic visions belong to the biblical and medieval tradition of apocalypse, of doom or final judgment. The link between doom and insanity preoccupied the Middle Ages as it preoccupies our own age. They saw the doom as foreordained; we see it as man-engendered. In every major period in history, writers and men of vision have felt this sense of doom. The prophet Daniel of the Old Testament, Gibbon of the eighteenth century, Huizinga of our own age and critics of the twentieth century such as Spengler have feared and analyzed declines and falls of civilizations. Many have argued that civilizations on the wane share certain characteristics. These include periods of revolution, both social and economic, the proliferation of new and often religious movements, increased interest in what the medieval theologians would have called "the pleasures of the flesh," a growth of religious enthusiasm and of mystical cults and, finally, an increased obsession with and manifestation of what has always been called "insanity."

The growth of medieval interest in insanity is manifest in twelfth-century literature, law, medicine and theology. Discussion of the subject reached a zenith in the fourteenth and fifteenth centuries, a period of decline in which death and madness were pervasive themes. To understand this period, we must examine the types of madness recognized by medieval men, and their treatments in the light of medieval medical, moral, legal and social sanctions. Here we shall find surprising legacies to our own world. The Arabs, for example, believed in the psychic origins of insanity and often treated it by a rudimentary form of psychotherapy, alternately agreeing and disagreeing with the patient so he would not take his fantasies too seriously. The modern world persists in ancient therapies and ancient attitudes: the economic circumstances of the madman and his observers did, as they do today, determine the diagnosis of his disease and the treatment he received.

As Greek, Roman and Judeo-Christian culture fathered the ideas of the Middle Ages, so the Middle Ages fathered the Renaissance, the beginning of the modern world, which, in turn, transmitted its ideals to us. Yet modern students, unlike medieval students, often suffer from the pride of present-mindedness. In the twelfth century, Chrétien de Troyes, the most influential writer of medieval romances, wrote in a preface to one of his "novels" that "chivalry passed from Greece to Rome and thence to France. God grant that it may remain here." He realized that the classical past was a direct ancestor, that it shaped his ideas. We might follow his example and recognize how much the Middle Ages has shaped our own ideas. This medieval influence is nowhere more evident in the modern world than in the definition and treatment of insanity.*

The history of the Western concept of thought is a progression from concern with the external forces to pre-occupation with the internal faculties. While the Greeks felt that the gods caused emotions, we in the modern world absolve our deities of the responsibility for our feelings and our actions. The medieval period stands between these two extremes. It marks a transition in the role of man from the victim to the guilty. Yet we have still to settle the questions of psychic responsibility. Is our psyche the product of our environment or of genetics? Is it pre-determined or changeable?

This book is dedicated to all students who wish to know what the adjective "medieval," so often used as a pejorative in psychiatry, should imply, and who want to become more aware of the historical formation of many concepts current in our lives.

---

* One case in point is Robert Burton's *Anatomy of Melancholy*. This seventeenth-century man of the modern world, in his analysis of mental disorder, cites classical sources, medieval sources and those classical sources specifically favored by medieval writers on the question of insanity.

# CHAPTER I

## THE PASSIONS OF THE SOUL
### Medieval Medicine and Psychiatry

> Madness cometh sometime of the passions of the soul . . .
>
> —BARTHOLOMEW OF ENGLAND

"In realizing its own rationality, mind also realizes the presence in itself of elements which are not rational."[1] These irrational elements may appear to dominate only the minds of madmen, yet, devoted as the twentieth century is to the reign of reason, it has often failed to recognize the irrational elements which shape conceptions and definitions of rational behavior.

The diagnosis and treatment of the extreme form of irrationality we call "insanity" are today, as they always were, determined by the biases of society. An aristocratic society is likely to perceive self-imposed poverty as a form of irrationality tantamount to insanity. For example, the king in a twelfth-century romance, seeing a knight strip himself of all his courtly vestments, associated nudity with derangement. The churchman of the Middle Ages, concerned less with economics and the niceties of custom than with sin and virtue, often saw madness as a punishment visited by God on the sinner. Medieval commentators tell us that Nebuchadnezzar was changed into a mad beast because of the bestial and irrational nature of his impieties. But the medical practitioners of ancient Greece, Rome and medieval Europe were, like modern doctors, interested in causes, symptoms and cures. Their concern was with those causes and cures of insanity which were explicable and treatable by empirical methods.

Aristocrats, clergy and doctors all agreed that madness was an "insania," a word which means an unhealth or what we call a disease and specifically a raving madness. They differed from one another in their conceptions of its origin and, as a consequence, of the effective treatment. But we can no more find any consistency in diagnosis and treatment among medieval doctors than we can in the modern medical establishment. Like modern psychiatrists, medieval physicians learned from the past and subscribed to a series of different medical theories of the origins, symptoms and treatments of diseases. Each of the various medieval therapies for the insane grew naturally out of a corresponding understanding of the origin of the disease. Cause, symptom and cure were linked to one another by the original sects of medical thought, but the Middle Ages was a period of synthesis. Eventually, the various medical theories of earlier authorities became intertwined with one another in a rich and varied eclecticism which was the legacy that the Roman court physician Galen and the second-century Cappadocian Aretaeus left to their medical successors.

Yet even in the eclectic medicine taught in the Middle Ages, it is possible to trace the distinctive traits of each earlier medical sect. Finally, each of these contributing sects left its mark, not only on the medieval theories but also on those of the centuries succeeding the Middle Ages. Even modern physicians who deny their diagnostic and therapeutic debts to the Middle Ages and its perpetuation of ancient ideas will recognize in these early definitions, diagnoses, symptoms and treatments of insanity the seeds of modern medicine.

Various medical schools of thought defined and treated insanity according to concepts which originated, not in medieval Europe, but in Greece, Rome and Byzantium. Four of the six great medical sects of the ancient world were of major importance in the medieval world. These were the humoral and the empirical sects of ancient

Greece and the pneumatic and eclectic sects of ancient Rome. Hippocrates' humoral theory was to survive the longest of the four, to dominate the study of human physiology and psychology for twenty-four centuries, but all four theories exercised a profound effect on medicine until the end of the seventeenth century. We, who still live in a world indebted to ancient medical theory, must consider the contributions and theories of each of these sects in order to understand the medical factors that determined the diagnosis and treatment of insanity.

## THE HUMORAL THEORY

Attempting to remove illness from the hands of the priests and the aegis of the gods, Hippocrates formalized the humoral theory of medicine based on the physical properties of the universe. Previous Greek philosophers had proclaimed a quadripartite structure of the universe. There were four elements: fire, air, earth and water. These four elements were analogous to four conditions. Fire was hot and dry; air was hot and moist; earth was cold and dry and water was cold and moist. Carrying these relationships a step further, Hippocrates isolated analogous substances in the human body and projected mental and physical states which arose from each. Blood, like air, was hot and moist and it promoted the rosy-cheeked face and the cheerful or sanguine temperament. Phlegm, like water, was cold and moist and its perceptible traits in man were a watery, colorless complexion and sluggish (phlegmatic) behavior. Black bile, generated in the liver, was cold and dry like earth. Its features were the dark, shaggy appearance and sad, solitary behavior of the melancholic (a word which means black bile). Yellow bile, a substance generated by the spleen, was hot and dry, and it produced the fiery-faced splenetic or choleric man. If it was burned by internal or external conditions of excessive heat, it became dark and was known as unnatural black bile, or adust melancholy, the psychic symptom of which was mania.

Hippocrates' principle accorded well with later, more anatomical medical theories which associated parts of the body and ages of life with the elements, the seasons of the year in which those elements prevailed and the various stars which ruled over these seasons. Humoral theory was transmitted to the West largely through Galen, whose own original contributions to medicine assured the survival of the Hippocratic traditions in which he also believed.

Seventeen hundred years after Hippocrates' death, Chaucer's physician had to know of "what humour" the patient's maladies were "engendered." Two centuries later still, in the Renaissance, Shakespeare, with his melancholy Dane and his seven ages of man, paid homage to the humoral theory. In the seventeenth century, Ben Jonson wrote *Every Man in His Humor* and Robert Burton dissected the "anatomy of melancholy." Much degraded, but strangely influential, the traditions survive to our day in the popular forms of horoscopes and words like "sanguine," "choleric," "manic," "phlegmatic" and "melancholic." The modern world is experiencing a resurgence of interest in the relations between genetics, birth seasons, physical traits and psychic dispositions. Once again we pursue a variant of the single most influential medical system of history.

## THE EMPIRICAL SECT

The empirical sect was a product of the anatomical school of Alexandria. According to this theory, the body had four vital organs—the brain, the heart, the spleen and the liver. If their shape, form or function was abnormal or impaired, the body, hence behavior, was likewise distorted. The most influential follower of this school was Constantine the African, an eleventh-century surgeon who taught at the medical school of Salerno, south of Naples, where he was the first to introduce the regular practice of surgery. His treatise on remembering and forgetting formalized for centuries the speculation of his theoretical predecessors that the brain had three parts, each of which performed a separate function.

> The operation of the mind is threefold. It is fantasy, rational intellect and memory. In the front ventricle of the brain, air is mixed and in that ventricle the animal spirit enters and makes the senses of sight, hearing, smelling, tasting, speech. From this space the animal spirit is carried to the medial ventricle where it is made pure and clearer for this is the seat of reason and intellect. The rear chamber is the seat of memory.[2]

For Constantine, the brain was the principal physical organ which affected the rest of the body and disorders resulted from its improper functioning. This was the opposite of the humoral theory. Hippocrates treated madness by restoring the physical balance of the humors: for too much melancholy (black bile), he gave food and drink to produce more blood which would compensate for the excesses of black bile. To deplete the liver's supply of bile, he offered the purgative herb hellebore. Constantine operated upon the brain, boring holes in it to clear a chamber of any obstruction. Constantine's system of brain function combined anatomy with an intangible force called "spirit," which can also be understood as air or force, what Bergson in the nineteenth century was to call "élan vital."

## THE PNEUMATIC SECT

Constantine's air or spirit was known technically as "pneuma," and he considered it the life-giving substance.

The groundwork for the belief that pneuma was the vital substance was first laid by Anaximenes, a Milesian philosopher of the sixth century before Christ. Until the first century before Christ, however, the pneumatic theories remained in an undeveloped state. Then a Greek physician from Cappadocia, Aretaeus, adapted some of the work of Hippocrates and developed a complex physiologic system, based upon a more fully developed concept of the predominance of pneuma in brain and body function. Although Aretaeus was most famous as the leader of the pneumatic sect, he was alive to the influence of other schools of medical thought and, as great synthesizers, he and his followers were the early innovators of eclecticism.

Aretaeus' most famous successor in the practice of pneumatic medicine was another Greek, Galen, who also practiced medicine in Rome. Galen advanced Hippocratic theories, but he combined them with a strongly anatomical orientation and produced that highly refined explanation of pneumatic function which was to be propounded by his most enthusiastic followers, the Arab physicians and philosophers who wrote and practiced from the eighth century through the twelfth. According to Galen, the pneuma was first mere air which, after it was inspired through the mouth, passed to the lungs, then moved to the heart. In the heart it was warmed and then moved in two parts and in two directions. A portion of the pneuma flowed downward and activated the lower organs of the body, where it operated as the "vital pneuma." Another portion moved upward and was purified in the brain, after which it became known as "psychic pneuma," the force controlling the noble and superior cerebral and spiritual functions.

Modern historians of psychology are aware that this invisible substance, pneuma, remained the most popular agent of transmission of impulses of the brain until Descartes proposed that fluid was the chief conductor. The current belief is that the impulses of the brain are electrical, and are transmitted by the nerve fibers and by substances known as neurohumors. The pneumatic school of medicine proposed some of the theories most attractive to some current psychiatric thinkers. Reichians and scientologists, for example, have transformed the pneuma into electrical energies which can be activated by the judicious application of electrical current. Mystical religions, particularly Oriental and communal cults, speak of concentrating our forces and of emitting electrical force fields. Even the Western concept of the divinity and intangibility of the mind is part of the heritage of pneumatic theory.

## THE ECLECTIC SECT

The major importance of the pneumatic school was not only its more abstract understanding of the human mind, but its contribution to the formation of a more flexible and holistic approach to psychiatry. Galen, who recognized the equal importance of pneuma, humors and anatomy, may be considered the first founder of eclectic medicine. He established the Western tradition of treating the mind and the body as parts of one whole. From his *Usefulness of the Parts of the Human Body*,[3] the later Arab proponents of an eclectic medicine learned to integrate their abstract, spiritual concept of the pneuma with anatomical discoveries. Out of their Galenic synthesis of pneuma, humors, anatomy, the Arabs forged a complex psychological theory which established them, rather than the Europeans, as the first true psychoanalysts. The Arabs and all who followed their course practiced a form of psychiatry resembling our own. They used abstract or intellectual cures which, however much they might utilize the body, worked principally on the brain. Doctors talked to the patient about his fears, and read to him from texts sprinkled with fallacies so that he could exercise his reason. They diverted him from concentrating on one sense by providing sensory antidotes, following the Arab theory that if one is haunted by dark fears, one should see bright and pleasant sights; if one is sad, one should hear happy music; and if one is in love and the lower parts of the body are too animated, one should exercise the upper portions of the anatomy by riding or playing ball. Today a similar reasoning is the foundation of anthroposophy, music, aversion therapy and milieu therapy.

The eclectic school was the product of the anatomical sects of Alexandria, the methodist sect of Soranus, the earliest humoral theories of Hippocrates and the pneumatic theories of Aretaeus and Galen. In Galen's greatest successors, we often see eclecticism. Though they might call themselves methodists or humoralists, medieval physicians, heavily influenced by the Arab theories which combined pneuma with anatomy, were unable to ignore the method of varied approach we call eclectic. At the height of its prominence, the medieval medical school at Salerno taught all of the major approaches to medicine. Its great surgeon, a monk from North Africa who adhered to the anatomical emphases of the Byzantines, Constantine, believed in the importance the methodist sect ascribed to the distance of atoms in the body, and in the principal importance of pneuma. Whatever he might call his sect, we would call him both an empiricist and an eclectic, and his influence on the concept of brain function remained primary for at least four centuries of European psychiatry.

In the eclecticism of the Middle Ages, the subtler forms of psychotherapy suggested by the earliest students of human nature flourished side by side with the more forthright physical treatments of surgery and shock, and each approach had its rationale. Byzantine doctors used psychic cures such as music therapy, playing cheerful tunes for the depressed and somber ones for the agitated. Roman therapists practiced a rudimentary form of electroshock therapy, using electric eels to treat depressed patients.

Both cures were a form of psychosomatic medicine, recognizing the interdependence of mind and body. The mind, refreshed by music, transmitted balanced and healthy impulses to the physiological system; the brain, its flesh jolted by current, restored proper spirit or thought. By further advancing this trend in ancient medicine, the Arabs made one of their most lasting medical contributions, as evidenced by this thirteenth-century English medical text, which is indebted to Arab sources:

> And so this animal spirit is gendered in the foremost den of the brain and is what spreads into the limbs of feeling: but nevertheless some part thereof abideth in the foresaid dens, that common sense, the common wit, and the virtue imaginative may be perfect. Then he passeth forth to the den of memory, and bearing with him the prints of likeness, which are made in those other dens, he layeth them up in the chamber of memory. From the hindermost parts of the brain he pierceth and passeth by the marrow and the ridge bone, and cometh to the sinews of moving, so that willful moving may be engendered in all parts of the nether body.
>
> . . . We may not believe that this spirit is man's reasonable soul, but more soothly, as saith Austin, the carrier thereof and proper instrument. For by means of such a spirit the soul is joined to the body; and without the service of such a spirit, no act the soul may perfectly exercise in the body.[4]

These are the major physiologic theories of the Middle Ages. For medieval physicians these theories determined the diagnosis and treatment of mental diseases. This entire corpus of psychological theory—humoral, pneumatic and, finally, eclectic—was disseminated by the great medieval medical school at Salerno.

## THE DISEASES OF THE MIND

By the ninth century Salerno was world-famous, revered as "the fountain of medical knowledge" and the "Civitas Hippocratica."[5] From East and West doctors came to practice and neophytes to learn medicine. North Africans, Frenchmen, Spaniards, Italians, Greeks—all of the literate world—learned medicine either at Salerno or, after its decline in the thirteenth century, at Montpellier in France. The causes and cures taught by these physicians spread throughout the medieval world, providing medieval physicians with a fairly homogeneous education. In order to graduate from Salerno, a student had to read Arabic, Hebrew and Latin. A knowledge of Hippocrates, Galen, Avicenna and Constantine was among the requirements for just one of the final examinations. Out of all the Greek, Roman and Arab approaches to medicine taught at Salerno, and later, after its decline, at Montpellier, grew the medieval concepts of disease.

By the ninth century, when Salerno had begun to be famous, medieval doctors had identified all of the major cerebral maladies. These they called stupor, phrenesy, epilepsy, hysteria, idiocy, mania and melancholy. The first four were physical diseases. Idiocy, an important social phenomenon, merited little attention in the medical texts, since it was designated both by law and by medicine as a permanent, hereditary state which was, consequently, intractable. Sophisticated physicians considered only mania and melancholy psychiatric problems.

As early as the seventh century, Isidore, bishop of Seville, and author of a monumental encyclopedia called the *Etymologies,* distinguished carefully between what he called "insania" (insanity) and "dementia" (mental deficiency, later called "amentia").[6] To Isidore, we owe not only the most precise medieval distinction between congenital idiocy and acquired insanity, but also the most thorough definition of the names of the two diseases generally considered acquired forms of insanity.

> *Mania* is named from insanity or "fury," because the ancient Greeks called fury *Manike* either from "unpropitiousness," iniquitas which the Greeks call Mania or from "divination" because the Greeks say *Manein* for "to divine." Black bile, *Melancholia,* is so named because it is a mixture of the dregs from black blood with an abundance of Bile. The Greeks call "Black" "Melas" and "bile" "Chole."[7]

Isidore called mania "a disordered state of mind characterized by fury and agitation, as distinguished from the depression . . . called melancholia [characterized by] disorientation, social withdrawals, and feelings of mistrust."[8] Isidore was concerned principally with the origins of the names of the diseases. In these origins, he found the causes of the diseases themselves. The first, mania, he saw as true insanity.* Melancholy was not insanity, at least in its initial stages, but arose from physical causes. It was lethargy which could develop into insanity. Even today it is easy to identify the man who raves and shrieks as "psychotic" while the man who withdraws or is constantly sad may be called a mere "depressive."

By the time of the flowering of Salerno, from the ninth century on, symptoms alone were insufficient evidence for identification of a maniac or a melancholic. Modern doctors differentiate among, for example, definitions, causes, clinical and laboratory manifestations, treatments and in-

---

* There is a quality of divinity in mania; the tradition that its agitation and raving were inspired was the legacy which the Dionysiac cults willed to the Western world. By the end of the Hellenistic period, the disease, like the gods who inspired it, had been degraded into insanity or, occasionally, by some churchmen, demonic possession by the old pagan gods who had become Christian demons.

cidence of disease. Medieval doctors at Salerno found it necessary to explain definitions, etiology, causes, effects and cures of disease, in the famous Salernitan book *On Chronic Diseases:*

> Mania and melancholy differ in place, material and effect, but they are made from the same humor. Mania is a disease affecting the anterior part of the brain [imagination and the senses] and melancholy is a disease affecting the middle part of the brain [reason or judgment]. The material of melancholy is natural melancholy [black bile]. The material of mania is unnatural melancholy [burned yellow bile]. The effect of mania is that it makes men enraged and that of melancholy is that it makes men timorous.[9]

Even a layman of the Middle Ages recognized the melancholic and the maniac by the symptoms they displayed. The maniac was fiery-complexioned, hyperactive, enraged, noisy and murderous. The melancholic was dark, shaggy, immobile, depressed, silent, solitary and suspicious. Mania was chronic, although the doctors did not abandon attempts at therapy; melancholy was temporary, but dangerous because it could be the first stage of mania. As early as the second century, Aretaeus recognized that syndrome which is now called manic depressive:

> And it appears to me that melancholy is the commencement and a part of mania. For in those who are mad, the understanding is turned sometimes to anger and sometimes to joy, but in the melancholic to sorrow and despondency only. But those who are mad are so for the greater part of life, becoming silly and doing dreadful things: but those affected with melancholy are not every one of them affected according to one particular form.[10]

Medieval doctors agreed that the insane showed insanity not only in their behavior but in their physical appearance. However, they disagreed on a central issue: Was the disease of madness primary or was it secondary? Did it originate in the brain and spread to the rest of the body or did it originate in the body and rise to the brain? Primary brain disease was, for example, brain fever or brain trauma. Secondary disease was often humoral imbalance.

## THE ORIGINS OF MADNESS

If the disease was primary, then the hope of cure was slight. It arose from two causes, either the passions of the soul or the introduction of excessive heat, cold, moisture or dryness into the brain. Each circumstance could affect either the first chamber of the brain, dulling its functioning senses and imagination, or the second chamber, blunting the reason and depriving the victim of judgment. Too much heat and dryness impaired the function of the vulnerable chamber, the senses and the imagination and produced a mania. Too much cold and dryness affected the chamber vulnerable to those conditions and the subsequent impairment of judgment resulted in melancholy. Prolonged continuation of these conditions eventually affected all the chambers of the brain, and the pathological conditions, as we might call them, moved along the traditional anatomical routes of the body, down to the spine, into the muscles and throughout the vital organs of the body, producing the physical symptoms of the disease. Bartholomew of England in the twelfth century cited those passions of the soul which were conducive to insanity: "[Madness comes] sometime of passions of the soul, as of busyness, of great thoughts, of sorrow and of too great study, and dread [and of] anger."[11] Here, in addition to the emotional extremes so feared by the Greeks and the medieval Arabs and Europeans, we find overactivity and profound concentration and study cited

as causes of madness, a sop to both the biblical and our
modern superstition that the intellectual is the man most
prone to insanity.

The secondary causes of insanity had already been
clarified by Hippocrates, for they were considered afflictions of the brain, arising in the disturbances of the body,
mainly humoral. An excess of black bile or of yellow bile
might rise to the brain, sometimes directly, sometimes in
the aurae or vapors associated with the pneumatic tradition. Black bile gravitated to the middle chamber, yellow bile to the foremost chamber. The etiology of these
afflictions is as complex as the body itself; black bile, produced by the liver, and yellow bile, produced by the
spleen and burned by heat (or passion or externally induced heat), became excessive under various conditions.
Diet, the ingestion of poison, weather conditions, the improper purgation of bile, urine, menses and sperm all
acted upon the liver, heart and spleen. To medieval doctors, diseases of the mind, when they were physically engendered, seemed to originate in some external cause,
weather or food, for example. The noxious substances collected or overproduced by these physical problems were
then carried either by the hypochondriac (stomach) region, in the case of flatulent melancholy, or by the blood
(especially in cases when heat thickened the blood), or
by the heart.

Each secondary cause of insanity carried its attendant
behavior, and Arnold of Villanova, a thirteenth-century
encyclopedist, wrote an elaborate description of the behavioral and delusional manifestations of each of the four
humoral types. It offers an excellent example of the medieval associations between etiology, symptoms and the
popular images in medieval delusions.

> If the affections are from the blood the signs are
> these: the patient laughs little all day and speaks in
> voices and in an hilarious manner and he wants to be

where musical instruments are beaten all day long. His blood is thick. If they proceed from choler he rages and is furious and angry; he shouts, jumps, runs and is wakeful and he has maniacal audacity; some assume the guises of animals and, unless they are restrained, they throw themselves out of the windows. . . .

If the affections come from phlegm the men are distracted, panicky and think that they are fish so that they want to look for water and to be in rivers or in the sea. This is from a humid complexion. . . .

If the passion is from melancholy the patient is worried and sad and he rouses the dead from their tombs. He believes that he is lying in his coffin, thinking himself a dead man; all day he weeps and has empty suspicions. Some think that they have no heads. Whence Galen said that he restored these to health with lead weights. Some believe that an angel supports the whole world and that, if he lets go, it will fall. Others hold their fists closed as if they were not able to open them, believing themselves in possession of a great treasure or believing that they hold the whole world in their fists and that it is subject to them. Some believe that they are vessels of clay and want no one to touch them, fearing lest they should break. They do not want others to look at them because they are afraid that they may be bewitched and immediately after spying them, they spit in clean places. Others extend their arms in the manner of cocks and, seeing cocks, they sing as if they were cocks, believing themselves to be so. Others fall into the worst suspicions, feeling love and hate for their relatives and they curse them.[12]

To any modern reader the signs and symptoms of what we call paranoia or schizophrenia are obvious. Only the forms they take vary from era to era. These particular

delusions are based upon and even portray genre scenes
of medieval life and they arise, according to this medieval
author, from physical, not supernatural sources. Yet even
the delusions reveal certain medieval assumptions: although there are angels they do not imitate Atlas; men
do not hold up the world; mad men are mad and not
bewitched; bewitchment can be a mere delusion.

Two spectacular forms of madness which we consider
peculiarly medieval delusions were love madness and
werewolfism or lycanthropy. In fact, they survived the
Middle Ages to haunt the imaginations of nineteenth-
century thinkers and writers and to be resurrected for
the delectation of twentieth-century moviegoers. Because
the nineteenth century considered them supernatural or
purely emotional in origin, twentieth-century popular
ideas hold that medieval men perceived them as demonic
in origin and sinister in effect. Medieval men believed, on
the contrary, that both of these diseases were natural in
origin and treatable by medical means.

The first, werewolfism, was universally recognized as a
disease which was humoral in origin. The Arabs, who discussed the well-known and, apparently, widespread disease most thoroughly and frequently in their treatises,
were divided on the issue of whether the disease was
melancholic or maniacal. However, physicians understood
that what began as a melancholy could develop into a
mania. By means of this argument, some of the opposing
opinions could sometimes be reconciled. Certainly, the
werewolf displayed a broad range of contradictory symptoms. He was dark, shaggy and hid himself in dark,
gloomy solitudes of graveyards and he displayed "lupinosity" and an "aspect not at all like that of a man."[13] Thus
he looked like a melancholic, but he also exhibited two
other symptoms which were maniacal: rage and a tendency to leap about.

Werewolfism was discussed at length by the greatest
encyclopedist of the thirteenth century, Vincent, bishop

of Beauvais.* Citing the Arabs Rhazes and Haly Abbas as his source, Vincent called the disease "canine melancholy," but other doctors called it "lupine mania." The only general point of agreement among all medical theorists and practitioners was the behavior of those afflicted with this malady. "They go about during the night imitating wolves in all things, and lingering around sepulchres till morning. They are pale, their vision feeble, their eyes dry and tongue very dry, and the flow of saliva is stopped; but they are thirsty and their legs have incurable ulcerations from frequent falls."[14]

Sometimes the doctors argued that, because the rage and hyperactivity displayed by them were symptoms of mania, the lycanthrope was a maniac. A fourteenth-century English physician, Bernard of Gordon, says, "If the disease which affects the patient arises from too much choler (yellow bile), we call it mania and the symptoms are leaping, rage, and lupinosity with a terrible mien. And those who have it are called daemones *lupini*."[15] On the other hand, the solitary fear of the werewolf is a melancholic symptom and some doctors called the disease "melancholia canina." Whoever was so transformed by his disease that his face was, as a Salernitan document tells us, "not at all like that of a man," was a werewolf. The disease was humoral in origin. If the offending humor was natural melancholy or black bile, the werewolf was a melancholic; if the offending humor was unnatural melancholy or burned yellow bile, the werewolf was a maniac, but medieval medicine never countenanced the belief that a man could actually change into a wolf. The doctor observing the afflicted man identified the offending humor by observing the behavior of the inhuman-looking

* Vincent was interested in the whole world of which the Bible was a part and the Bible described the first werewolf, Nebuchadnezzar. Vincent, however, restrained his moral tendencies and confined his examination largely to the physical nature of the disease as it was known to the doctors.

creature. Then he decided how to expel or counteract the excess of yellow or black bile.

The second disease, love madness, was for medieval men, indisputable in its origins. It was always melancholic in nature. Known as "amor heroicus," or erotic love, love madness was mentioned by Hippocrates, Galen and all of those later physicians who renewed their knowledge of it through Arab medical documents. It too survived into the nineteenth century, when people "died of broken hearts."

There were two schools of thought about the origin of the disease. It could come from physical causes, the damming up of the sexual secretions and other substances presumably released by coition. It could arise from psychic causes, obsession with the beloved which caused the damming up and overproduction of bile. In either case, the symptoms of the lovesick man or woman had serious physical consequences and could result in death. Although we no longer think of lovesickness as a genuine disease, we can still recognize the symptoms medieval physicians described, since we still believe in the same "signs of the lover."

Their eyes are hollow, and do not shed tears, but appear as if overflowing with gladness; their eyelids move rapidly; and even when none of the other parts of the body are affected, these parts are always so affected in lovers. There is no pulse peculiar to lovers, as some have supposed, but it is the same as that of persons laboring under care. When they call to recollection the beloved object, either from seeing or hearing, and more especially if this suddenly occurs, then the pulse undergoes a change from the disorder of the soul, and, therefore, it does not preserve its natural equability or order. [They are] desponding and sleepless.[16]

Again, doctors were in agreement on the symptomatic definition of the disease and they closely followed the Arab treatises. Arnold of Villanova offers the most inclusive and concise definitions of the disease, omitting its etiology, and quoting an influential Arab definition: "Amor Heroicus is the sensual desire of one individual human being of one sex to embrace the individual of the other sex, which is commonly called love and, by the doctors, erotic, boundless and irrational love."[17] This irrational, unconsummated love could develop into a melancholia. Those physicians who adhered to the belief that the disease was a primary affliction of the brain, a more romantic and, hence, more modern view of the disease, called love "an affection of the brain since it consists of certain cares," and maintained that care was "a passion of the soul occasioned by the reason's being in a state of laborious emotion."[18] This love was one of those melancholies from interior causes which had to be physically treated by amusement, spectacles, diversions or reunions with the beloved. The practical Arab and the moral Christian view of love madness coincided nicely as the first sought to alleviate the passions of the flesh and the second to condemn them. For both love madness was the result of sexual frustration, brought on by obsession with the person of the beloved. It was caused by "too much wakefulness, and from the retention of the blood which used to flow out through the nostrils and through the hemorrhoids or owing more to the retention of the menses or corrupted sperm or through any other kind of retention and this, as we have seen, often happens to the spouseless religious men and women, for, as Galen said, sperm which is retained more than it should be, is converted into poison."[19] Such poisons rose to the brain on aurae or vapors from the liver, the medieval seat of love, and the organ which produced black bile or melancholy. A disease so caused can be cured only by proper purgation of sperm and menses, a treatment highly recommended by

Chaucer's wife of Bath, by several of the medieval Tristan figures and even by some popular theorists and pamphleteers in the twentieth century. In 1972, a French schoolteacher was condemned for exposing her students to a recent pamphlet which proclaimed the necessity of purging and exercising the sexual organs for the maintenance of mental and physical health.

Whatever the origin, whether in blood or liver, heart or spleen, whether from food or poison or weather conditions or excessive emotion, the diseases of both melancholy and mania, if neglected, became firmly entrenched and pervaded the whole brain and body system of man. Medieval doctors called a "compound mania" or "melancholia," a mania or a melancholia in which all the chambers of a person's brain and all the vital organs and the blood were flooded with the substances of his disease. Then he was a man caught in a vicious mind-body cycle.

## THE THERAPIES

The eclecticism of most medieval physicians motivated them to practice different types of therapy, but each disease was treated on the basis of its etiology and the practitioner's adherence to the therapy prescribed by the medical "sect" he embraced. For example, the physician who devoted his attention to the humors might believe that the origin of a patient's mania was an overheating or excess of the blood. He would treat the disease by attempting to cool the hot blood with cooling substances like white wine or by draining off the excess blood through cupping or venusection. If, however, the physician concluded that the mania was caused by turbulent emotions which consequently overheated the brain, he treated the emotions. The psychotherapeutic measures available to him were conversation, lessons in reason or logic, the provision of relaxing activities and settings and narcotics.

The major treatments in use were remarkably all-inclusive. Physicians practiced herbal therapy, diet therapy, hydrotherapy, physiotherapy, surgery and psychotherapy. The Arabs, tracing some of their practices to Dioscorides, were particularly adept in the use and preparation of drugs which they referred to as "lettuces" and "poppies," and which we would call opiates. In this chemotherapy, also called herbal therapy, the first general use of tranquilizers is apparent. More conservative physicians abhorred the violent effects of some of the drugs and prescribed, instead, therapeutic diets. Diets were designed either to counteract the offending humor (for example, red wine produced more blood to balance black bile or warm the cold melancholic) or to purge the body of an excess of humoral fluid through the use of either emetics or laxatives.

Physiotherapy in the form of lower-body exercises for the problems of erotic obsession is a common recommendation in Arab texts. Vincent of Beauvais, taking up the Arab recommendations in his later work, suggested games of ball and cold showers for erotomania. Warm baths were prescribed for relaxing and moistening the hot, dry maniac. The anatomically oriented successors of the Byzantine theorists sometimes practiced brain surgery on the principle that trepanning, or incising of the skull, would permit compressed atoms of flesh to move apart and thus relieve the pressure on the brain which they believed was causing these operable cases of insanity. Results could verify the treatment, for those patients who survived the operation sometimes emerged symptom-free of the disease. Medical historians have concluded that those cured patients had been suffering from brain tumors and that the pressure of the tumor had been relieved by the opening in the skull.

The more psychoanalytically oriented cures have the cast of modernity. The Byzantines, for example, had recommended and used music therapy. They even codified the musical modes or scales effective in the cures of

various diseases. The martial, orderly Doric mode imposed
sobriety and self-control on the maniac. The cheerful
Ionian mode would gently enliven the melancholic. The
most sophisticated methods of psychotherapy were none
of these, nor were they tinged by the superstition which
permitted some physicians to rub patients' heads with
balms or apply the pulverized heart of a stag. We recognize in them variations on our own milieu therapy, play
therapy and psychoanalysis.

Many Arab physicians urged that the melancholic be
placed in pleasant, cheerful settings, and advised the pursuit of interesting diversions such as hunting or riding.
Most amazing is their sophistication in psychoanalytic in-
tervention. They argued that the patient should be removed from all false examinations and questions, that he
should be exposed regularly to calming reason and that
his fears, although they should not be indulged or encouraged, should be discussed. Their sophistication and
humaneness is a source of modern amazement and delight.

When all other cures failed, prayer and the preparation of magic talismans and charmed ointments might be
tried. Contrary to current popular opinion, however, the
trained physicians did not rely exclusively on either magic
or religious help. Such cures do appear in fiction, as they
did in real life, but their province was not chiefly medical.
Medical schools did not teach the preparation of charms
or demonology. Nevertheless, at two points, medieval
medicine crosses and combines with astrology and theology. These are the hereditary predisposition to disease
and the universal philosophical concept of balance and
order in the universe. God predetermined both, in the
medieval view, and with this fixed, divine order, even the
physicians had to deal.

## PREDISPOSITION AND HEREDITY

Even before his birth, the medieval man was predestined, not only to salvation or damnation in the afterworld, but also to illness or health, sin or virtue, strength or weakness in this world. Chaucer's physician, like any good doctor of his century, could predict his patients' problems by consulting the stars. True, he applied to his treatments and prognoses a form of magic called "natural magic" which was sometimes condemned by churchmen, but his methods were nevertheless often used by many of these same clerics when they were trained in the theory and practice of medicine. At birth, each man or woman was predisposed, not by genes but by the circumstances of his birth, to a physical constitution inextricably intertwined with an accompanying personality. The determining force was astrology, the conjunction of stars and planets in the zodiac at the time of the patient's birth.

Proof of the generality of this belief and its application to the practice of medicine appears repeatedly in charts, diagrams and aphoristic poems of the period. Many of these documents constitute an important part of the literature taught at medieval medical schools. A Salernitan mnemonic poem teaches the student the proper relation between the constellations and the portions of the body over which they exercise control.

For Aries rejoices to have under its control the
    head and face;
Power over the throat and neck is given to Taurus.
The arms with the hands are, appropriately enough,
    dominated by the Gemini;
Cancer rules the depths of the breast.
Leo claims the stomach and both kidneys.
And Virgo claims preeminence over the intestines.
Libra controls both buttocks and the ribs.

Scorpio has exclusive power over the anus and the
 pudenda.
Sagittarius holds sway over the hips;
Capricorn rules both knees.
Under the rule of Aquarius, appropriately, fall both
 legs;
With Pisces are the soles of the feet exclusively
 in accord.[20]

Personality was determined, then, by the star under which
a man was born and by the interaction of that star with
the planets both at the time of birth and ever after. The
seasons also mediated in man's physical and psychological
fate. The Salernitan treatise on the four humors, relying
heavily upon the Hippocratic work *Airs, Waters and
Places,* correlates the four elements, the four seasons, the
four ages of man and the four temperaments, and the
picture is far bleaker than that depicted by Shakespeare
in his remarks on the seven ages of man, written four
centuries later.

Air, blood, childhood and spring are consonant
 with one another;
Fire, summer, choler and youth are in accord;
Autumn, earth, melancholia and old age,
Decrepitude and winter, water and phlegm are all
 bound to each other.[21]

Medieval men often saw both sin and illness as imbal-
ances, the results of physical and emotional excess. The
path of philosophical virtue became the route to mental
health.

In the works of a popular German homeopathist, the
tenth-century nun Hildegard of Bingen, we see some of
the ingenious ways in which sin and madness, theology
and medicine, became intertwined into a form of psychiatry which cannot be explained by physiology alone. For

even the physiologists, God was the ultimate source of all health. In Hildegard's words, the devil works not directly on man's soul, but through his body, on his soul. Hildegard should be the patron saint of any work on medieval madness, since for her, melancholy is the original disease.

For Adam knew good, and, by eating the apple, he committed a sin. As the actual change took place, melancholy rose up in him, which is not in man, awake or asleep, without the suggestion of the devil. As a result of his transgression, Adam felt sadness and despair because of melancholy. At the very moment that Adam disobeyed the divine ordinance, melancholy became an integral part of his blood just as splendor departs when a light is extinguished and just as burning flax leaves behind a foul smoke. And so it was in Adam because, when the splendor was extinguished, melancholy was coagulated in his blood from which sadness and despair rose up in him.[22]

# CHAPTER II

## THE DEATH OF NOBILITY
*Insanity and the Medieval Church*

> When a man loses his reason, he dies,
> since the noblest thing in him dies.
>
> —LUCIAN

"She has a devil within her, and may God restore her to her right mind." This outcry against madness as demonic possession was heard during the Middle Ages, but it never had the universal currency that present-minded men of the twentieth century would like to imagine. Yet, for many today, demonic possession remains the simplest, the most dramatic and, secretly, the most attractive of all explanations of insanity in the Middle Ages. Perhaps we revel in the exposure of a primitivism and superstition which the catchall phrase reveals. Perhaps we are moved by the exciting and terrifying descriptions of the experts on demonology, the medieval churchmen. Certainly, the directness and color of the ritual cure, exorcism, have a broad appeal; since the possessed acted "mad," they had to be distinguished from the insane.

The behavior of the possessed man or woman was immediately recognizable. He could not pray; he could not take the eucharist, for he would vomit it out. He could not calmly behold the image of Christ. He raved, but his ravings were those of the madman, for he was, as we say, "not himself," because the devil had literally taken possession of him. Before the priest could cure the demoniac, he had to identify him, and he did so, not only by his behavior, but also by his appearance. A composite account drawn from the Bible and the writings of the early clerics offered the exorcist a picture identical to that of the unclean spirits healed by Christ in the Gospels.

Demoniacs have faces which hardly resemble human beings: Their lips are drawn tight and their mouths work as if manipulated by another. Frequently, the lips are stretched taut in a hideous grimace while foam gushes from between their teeth. A noxious stench seems to leak from their pores. Their eyes roll in their heads, so that they seem now to be blind, now to be fixed in a piercing and unnatural stare. Their mouths belch forth curses and obscenities. Their limbs are contorted and jerk spasmodically, and they are often thrown to the ground by a force not their own. When they do speak, they speak with the voice of another. They are wasted by their ordeals, yet usually unable to eat. Worst, they abhor the name of God and the sight of his symbols.

Anyone into whom the devil had entered behaved like a raging madman. The Greeks said that the possessed were driven by the Furies, the medieval Christians that they were impelled by the "unhealthy madness of sin." If the devil were not driven out, the demoniac could be the victim of a destruction just as devastating, but more visible than the ruin of his soul. A thirteenth-century bishop, Caesarius of Heisterbach, in his *Dialogue on Miracles*, left a startling description of the fate of one victim.

A certain noble lady of Saxony was grievously tormented by a devil who haunted her. Her servants, to restore her sanity, took her to various shrines of the saints and one day, a priest coming up, a man of mean appearance but endowed with the grace of God, felt pity for her torments. For out of his abounding charity, he besought the Lord and drove out the devil, restoring the woman to her right mind. But he charged her to receive the sacrament for thirty days whilst remaining in the same place, and to hear the services of the canonical hours for those days. After she had done it for nine days, her people, thinking it no harm, took her away. On the way she was struck by a great gust of wind, thrown down and so utterly dashed to pieces by the devil that all her limbs looked just like human entrails.[1]

Since demonic possession was a spiritual illness, no physical remedy could cure it. The priest and God were the only physicians, and the exorcists engaged in this spiritual medicine favored various methods for trapping and expelling the devil. Names were accorded a special curative power. The name of God was the most potent weapon against the devil, but the knowledge of the devil's name gave the priest the ability to summon and order his adversary. Often the exorcist directed some of his most forceful efforts to eliciting the name of the inhabiting devil, be it Asmodeus or Belial. By the seventeenth century, a standard and orthodox formula for exorcism was set forth in the *Rituale Romanum*. First the priest gathered his own powers by praying for inner peace, faith and confidence. Only when he felt that he had achieved these, could he proceed in his assault upon the devil. This he conducted by conjuring the unclean spirit, "the adversary of all," to come forth from the possessed. The demon was commanded "in the name of him who rules the seas and the winds, the heavens and the earth, in the name of him who was crucified for men," that he "go back to the regions from whence [he] came."[2] The crucifix was then applied to the forehead and later to the breast, then again to the forehead of the possessed, who heard that the curative powers rested not with the earthly exorcist, but with the heavenly God.

The skillful exorcists were men of extraordinary piety, those least bound to earth and, hence, to the weaknesses of worldliness. Of course, the saints, whose biographies were frequently modeled after the life of Christ, were famous for their acumen in dealing with the devil. The saints' talent for healing demoniacs was the result not only of their natural piety but also of their many trials with devils who apparently found such virtue challenging. The most popular and widely circulated medieval compilation of saints' lives was the *Golden Legend* by Jacobus de Voragine, a Dominican preacher of the thirteenth century. His life of St. Augustine illustrates a well-known fact: saints might be continually tempted by the devil, but they never succumbed to him, so they were never possessed.

According to Jacobus, saintly piety could enrage the devil himself. One day St. Augustine saw the devil pass by carrying a book which, he told Augustine, contained the sins of man. Asking to see the place where his own sins were recorded, Augustine discovered that the page was empty except for a notation that he had once forgotten compline (late night services). Augustine went immediately to recite compline with much devotion and then returned to scan the devil's page, which he now found completely blank. In a rage, the devil ranted that he had been deceived because the saint had wiped out his sin through prayer. Here prayer was a talisman against diabolic power. In Jacobus' legend of St. Martin, faith and steadfastness fend off the deceiving devil. St. Martin was besieged by the devil, who appeared first in the form of Mercury, then in the form of Jupiter and, last, in the guise of a king who declared he was Christ. When Martin announced that he would not believe that he saw Christ until he saw him in the attire of the crucifixion and bearing the stigmata, the devil vanished and the air was filled with his stench.[3]

The insight and fidelity of a saint imbued with the instinct for divinity might save him from the clutches of evil, but the less-gifted were all too often deceived. Then these unfortunate sinners needed the services of the saintly. Prayers and exorcising formulas were the most effective means of driving out the devil, but they were not the only methods available. The laying on of hands, usually practiced in cases of physical illness, was also used against devils, as were the magic talismans, the book and the crucifix and the eucharist itself. Most attractive to medieval believers was faith healing, and tales of the curative miracles performed by saints abounded. The medieval demoniac whose local priest could not help him might be led to the nearest appropriate shrine.

Certain saints were considered particularly effective against possession and its attendant insane behavior. Today, the shrines and churches of these saints are still highly regarded as therapeutic sites, principally for the cure of the mad. The modes by which many saints became associated with the cure of madness are fascinating because of the literal and simple reasons for the attribution of their powers. St. Front of Périgueux became a saint of the mad merely because of his name, which is the same as the French word for forehead. His martyrdom and his special gifts had nothing to do with insanity. St. Symphorien, after whom numerous churches in France are named, was beheaded for refusing to worship Venus. Visitors to his shrines sought cures for all diseases of the head. The most famous psychiatric saint, Dympna, an Irish princess of the year 600, was credited with resisting the incestuous advances of her father, who pursued her to the Continent and beheaded her. Her shrine at Gheel in Belgium, where she was reportedly buried, was for centuries the favored site for the cure of demoniacs. To this day, Gheel is a town reserved for the mad, who are housed there in individual and homelike domiciles.

By whom and how demonic possession can be recognized and cured is not merely a question of the dark past. The current interest in such popular works as William Peter Blatty's *The Exorcist* attests to the vitality of modern concern with devils and demonic possession in popular as well as ecclesiastical circles. Blatty's young Jesuit psychiatrist consults with scholarly avidity the works of authorities in the exorcist's manual, canon law and especially the modern classic on possession, *Possession: Demoniacal and Other*, written by the German scholar T. K. Oesterreich in 1921. Before he can treat the heroine of the novel, he must ascertain whether he is confronting a genuine case of possession, a hypnotic state, a case of hysteria or one of schizophrenia. Only true possession can be treated by an exorcist. The others are recognized today, as they were by the learned in the Middle Ages, as forms of mental illness susceptible to psychotherapy and drug therapy.

Yet the history of the confusion between forms of possession and forms of insanity is a long one. A number of cultural historians have pointed to the resemblance between states of shamanistic or ecstatic trance and modern hysteria.[4] The figures in whom they have found these confusing behaviors range from the pythoness, oracle of Delphi, to the Corybantes, the Dionysiac celebrants, to an apparently possessed Carmelite nun of the twentieth century, Marie Thérèse Noblet.[5] In these and other prophetic and eccentric figures the historians find the same rolling of the eyes, the same oblivion after each ordeal, the same contortions of the limbs as those observed in clinical studies and descriptions of confirmed hysteria. The skeptic and modern rationalist will see, in all these cases, schizophrenia or hysteria. Yet contemporary men of faith, particularly those within the church who follow the orthodox traditions, remain convinced that demonic possession is a real and present phenomenon which we must not confuse with the purely psychic conditions we call psychoses.

In a study entitled *True and False Possession*, the French neurologist Jean LHermitte wrote in 1963 that he could not evade the question so often put to him, "Do you really believe in the existence of demoniacal possession?" He replies, "As a Christian, I can only answer that I do." He says that a modern physician will find "in the woman bent double, a paralytic, in the biblical energumen of Gerasa, a madman, and in the boy cured on the morrow of transfiguration, an epileptic."[6] LHermitte warns that both psychic and physical disturbances may be either natural or caused by the devil and that physicians may indeed treat the former diseases, but that theologians alone are qualified to treat the latter.

LHermitte despairs of the efforts of modern physicians. Jesus alone, he believes, was gifted with an infallible and instinctive certainty about the differences between sickness and demonic possession. Modern readers, he insists, can find proof of this talent in the Bible, for Jesus merely touches the sick, but he exorcises the possessed by calling forth the inhabiting devil. His book is written to offer less-gifted men the guideposts they need to help them perceive the differences between genuine and pseudo diabolic possession. The establishment of these criteria was one of the goals of T. K. Oesterreich's earlier study.

Oesterreich cited three incontrovertible signs of possession. These were the alteration of the physiognomy, the alteration of the voice and, most important, the substitution of a new and alien ego, a fact proved by the demoniac's knowledge of events and languages to which he had not been privy during his life. Surveying all the major varieties of possession from those found among the ancient Egyptians to those found among the Greeks, the medieval Christians and, finally, those apparent in modern French and German cases, Oesterreich found two major types. These were spontaneous possession, in which the man or woman possessed was simply overtaken by the possessing spirit, and voluntary possession, a state deliberately induced or even contracted for by a person desirous of union with another spirit. Sometimes the possessed was unconscious of his state and had no memory of it after it had ended, a form Oesterreich calls somnambulistic possession. Sometimes he is lucid and retains a clear impression of his experience after it has terminated. Noting that a person can be possessed by spirits other than the devil, Oesterreich lists, among the invaders, the spirits of the living or the dead and the spirits of animals.

In the Middle Ages, Oesterreich discovers frequent cases of zoanthrophy and cynanthropy, states in which the people affected believed that they were animals and especially wolves or dogs. Acting out their new roles, they took refuge in forests, grew long hair and nails, attacked and ate children and behaved like wild animals. These he does not consider cases of "true possession." The differentiating factor was the general permanence of these animalistic trances and the temporary or fitful nature of true possession. Actually, the literature of the Middle Ages belies his view, since, in fiction, the werewolves returned to human form and, in Arab medical treatises, lycanthropy was a humoral disease, subject to the cures for excessive black or yellow bile. More accurately, the author concludes that possession during the "Christian Middle Ages" was demonic, whereas modern possession, in which he was a firm believer, is affected principally by the spirits of the dead. This fact indicates to him a modern decline of faith in the devil and demonology in general, a conclusion with which the readers of the seventies would certainly not concur.

Possession was a common enough threat in the Middle Ages to be the subject of much discussion and debate. As strong as the force of God was, so strong was the force of the devil. Some theologians believed that the devils, not satisfied with merely tempting men, needed their bodies for warmth and, in a constant search for a source of heat, would enter the mansion of human flesh whenever they could, by overpowering those human forces for goodness which naturally excluded demonic invasion. Some believed that people, falling into sin, actually invited the visitation of the devil through the abandonment of their wills which fought against sin. Yet, because the medieval world was beset with devils, the most brilliant minds of the age evolved a series of complex explanations for the birth and flowering of evil in the universe and in the souls of men.

These explanations were the province of the theologians whose doctrines pervaded medicine, law, morality and popular belief. Such doctrines affected the educated because the teaching of reading, writing, medicine, law, music, rhetoric and philosophy was a church monopoly. The educators were all clerics, a word which means a learned man or a teacher. They affected the populace, who were treated by church-trained doctors and were taught morality and faith by priests. The popular opinion of the Middle Ages we cherish is fully cognizant of the influence of the church, but it fails to take into account the fact that many of the churchmen also had allegiances to physiology, to law and to poetry, all of which might be influenced by theology but were not necessarily overwhelmed by it.

Isidore of Seville in the seventh century and Vincent of Beauvais in the thirteenth were both bishops, yet in their encyclopedias they chose to study geography, medicine and history. Constantine was a monk, yet he practiced surgery at the medical school of Salerno. Although all of these men shared interests in the doctrines of good and evil, they also professed other crafts and trades with attendant philosophies. No sophisticated ecclesiastic could content himself with the belief that "simple demonic possession" explained all of human behavior, and even if all believed in the influence of the devil, the nature of that influence could be complex indeed. For these reasons, if the influence of church doctrine in the Middle Ages cannot be overemphasized, its concepts should not be oversimplified.

The paths and powers of the devil were subtle and ubiquitous. Under his aegis, sin, injustice, famine and disease of all kinds flourished. He played his role in insanity as he played his role in every illness and misfortune, but medieval theologians, lawyers and physicians made clear distinctions between insanity and possession. Insanity might follow from possession or possession from insanity, but they were not identical, merely associated. The link between them was the destruction of order in the universe and the individual. Nowhere is the relation between reason and the devil better exemplified than in a tale of the *Gesta Romanorum*, the most popular medieval storybook of ancient tales, which were moralized, allegorized and written down in the fourteenth century. The plot of the instructive tale is simple, the moral complex. A child was attacked by a serpent. A greyhound sleeping near the child was roused by the attack and fought the snake. In the course of the battle, the greyhound was wounded, but he saved the child. The allegorization of the tale explains that the greyhound is reason and the serpent is the devil. The moral is that reason, as soon as it is stirred from the sleep of sin, fights the devil, but the devil wounds reason as often as he brings a man to life willfully and not by reason. The conclusion of the tale is that, when his reason is asleep, a man is easy prey for the devil and that conclusion is sufficiently prevalent in the Middle Ages to warrant an examination of the meaning of reason in the medieval world.

## REASON

Reason is the single most important philosophical principle in the cosmology of the Middle Ages. Its meaning is so all-encompassing, its influence so great that it was the foundation of all the moral and theological explanations of man's physical and spiritual being which, when healthy, were called his "sanity." When a man suffered a privation or a serious disturbance of his reason, he was considered unhealthy and demented, "insanus." No theologian could properly understand God, the nature of the world or the human mind without first understanding the meanings, genesis and process of reason. In the literatures of the age, "reason," *ratio* in Latin, is the word which is perhaps richest in its multiplicity of meanings.

According to St. Augustine and his followers, the Bible proclaimed that God is reason. He is, as the Gospel of St. John said, "logos." Augustine believed that God gave a portion of that reason to men and that this rich legacy is what makes man divine and raises him above the beasts. The text which Augustine cites to prove this theory is the passage from Genesis asserting that "God created man in his own image." The image of God, the church fathers said, was reason. They do not intend that we should interpret this reason as the mere faculty of cerebration. Reason, in this sense, is to be understood as order, stability and a quality of the soul inherent in that instinctive kind of wisdom which attracts men to goodness and repels them from evil. Loss of reason is loss of the instinct for virtue. As the immortal and eternal principle of order, reason was also considered a quality of man's immortal portion, the soul.

Elaborating upon the Platonic doctrine of soul and reason, the early church father Tertullian recalled Plato's division of the soul into rational and irrational elements. He pointed out that, at the time of creation, God imbued man's soul with reason and concluded that, for this reason, we should regard as natural to the soul "that rational element which was implanted in it at the beginning, namely by its rational author."[7] Irrationality, then, was considered a denial of the Creator and a loss of the most natural part of the soul itself. Yet reason came to be associated with the narrower function of judgment, located in the central chamber of the brain.

Although some societies located reason in the heart and others in the head, all came to associate it with the faculties of the mind. This was largely due to St. Augustine's conclusion that God, who was order, wisdom and reason, had endowed man with a mind capable of some of that reason so that he would worship his source. Highest of faculties, the reason or mind was in the head, the organ nearest God. "But there is a third thing," argues St. Augustine, "the head, as it were, or the eye of our soul or whatever else more fitly describes reason and intelligence, which beasts do not have. Can you, I pray, find anything in human nature higher than reason?"[8] In Colossians, Paul had located reason, however metaphorically, in the head, but this was the head of the angels as well as the head of men. He proclaimed that in Jesus "dwelleth all the fulness of the Godhead bodily. And you are complete in him which is the head of all principality and power."[9] Ultimately, by grace of anatomy, philosophy and theology, rationality became a property of the human mind. It was this property which symbolized health, wholeness and virtue. Irrationality, in its extreme form insanity, became a malfunction of the link between man and God.

With the physicians, the theologians shared the conviction that reason was the purest faculty of the brain and of the soul and that it controlled all the functions of the human body. The very fact that reason did reside in the head or in the brain was, however, dangerous to its survival. Flesh was visible, changeable, corruptible. Flesh rebelled against will and destroyed reason. The mansion of the body entertained the destruction of the mind it housed. The world of physical objects and flesh was visible but blind. If men heeded the call of the flesh instead of the call of reason, they were sinners and no better than animals who lived by blind instinct alone.

For both pagans and Christians, the soul and the mind faced their worst adversary in the body. It was the body which erred, the body which desired, the body which decayed. "And were we not saying long ago that the soul when using the body as an instrument of perception, that is to say, when using the sense of sight or hearing or some other sense—were we not saying that the soul too is then dragged by the body into the region of the changeable and wanders and is confused: the world spins about her and she is like a drunkard when she touches change?"[10]

These are the words of Socrates, who mistrusted the body and praised the soul. So did such later Christians as Boethius, who maintained that the farther one lived from God, and earth was the sphere farthest from God, the more unstable and inaccurate was the motion of the sphere and life itself. Man, it seems, by dint of his distance from God, his dependence on the senses, his embodiment in flesh, was doomed to instability and irrationality and yet he was gifted by God with reason. This problem deeply troubled the fathers of the church, who spoke not in terms of insanity, but of irrationality.

The world began with the end of chaos, banished by the principle of reason and order which "was God and was with God." St. Augustine argued that an infinitely good God created a world which was perfect because it was the embodiment of all the godly qualities of measure, form and order, which define goodness. There was no evil at creation, nor, St. Augustine said, did God create evil. Man was endowed with the goodness of the universe, order and reason. Yet man also had the potential to sin because he had desires and was capable of concupiscence, fleshly desire, which he controlled by the exercise of his God-given will. Human irrationality is really postlapsarian, and man is responsible for its appearance in the world, for, according to St. Augustine's doctrine of free will, man had and has the ability to choose any course of action he wishes. God may know what course a man may choose but he never interferes directly in that choice. So, by the free submission of his will to desires and appetites, to the flesh, Adam brought disorder and irrationality into the world. The natural consequence of this belief was that irrationality, the extreme form of which is insanity, is a turning away from God or reason and is, for that reason, impious. Only the sinful would reject divine order and reason, which God had implanted within them.

Although few of the theories we have so far discussed emphasize the role of the devil in the world, there were many theologians who shared more than a suggestion of St. Augustine's early Manichaeism. They believed that the devil and God were at war, forever embattled in a conflict of which the chief prize was the soul of man. One of the most ingenious variations of this theme is the philosophy of the nun Hildegard of Bingen. She combined a belief in the devil with an interest in physiology, and the issue of this marriage was her theory that sin was an unhappy coincidence of physiology and diabolic temptation. A temperament prone to insanity is the legacy of all men born after Adam's submission.

In medical treatises of the era insanity was caused not only by the destruction or corruption of reason but also by the impairment of the imagination or the senses or by excessive production of a bodily humor which rose to the brain. We see in the examination of church philosophy the moral elevation of abstract reason or wisdom to such a height that the senses are viewed as either positive evils or unfortunate but necessary implements for obtaining a glimpse of wisdom. The senses, and the imagination, when they are treated by the church philosophers, are too frequently discussed in pejorative tones. They are the body and the body decays. Our flesh makes us heirs to temptation and sin; our senses deceive us and our organic necessities pollute the pure spirit, air, and the incorporeal nature of reason. If man was created "a little lower than the angels," then his senses were lower than his reason and his flesh was lower still.

Yet the flesh was not considered despicable by all. Some said that we should understand the passage "God made man in his own image" as a statement that God too was made of earth. All agreed that the flesh, at creation, was not evil, since God "saw that it was good." Nevertheless, the flesh could be the devil's portal if it turned inward upon itself. If it turned toward God it was precisely what God intended it to be: a mansion for the rational soul, a receptor of information which could warn the soul to shun sin. Yet, in the mouths of the fathers, these arguments ring hollow. Like our celebrations of the flesh today, those treatises seem to be protesting too much that the "body too has its place," that we must remind ourselves not to condemn the physical as "merely physical."

In the fourteenth century and afterward, the plague and the *fin de siècle* mood which provoked the dance of death and the literature of mortification, we find both less reticence to condemn the body as a stinking tomb and more extravagantly riotous celebrations of the joys of hedonism. But, until that time, we share with the Middle Ages the puritanism which condemned the flesh. Skin, bones and vital organs were the weakest portions of humankind and were, in their vulnerability and mortality, the vehicles of temptation. Shakespeare called the body "heir to a thousand ills" and madness was considered one of those ills. For the medieval physician, theologian and, perhaps even more, the ordinary man, madness was, as it is today, the most pernicious and terrifying of all "diseases." The horror and even the purpose of insanity in particular cannot be understood without a primary exposure to the purely theological and moral explanations of disease in general.

## DISEASE

The fall, generally considered the first moment at which disease and the imperfections of man's mind and body entered the world, was not seen as the last. In all the events of human history, theologians saw a reflection of the divine scheme of rewards and punishments. No human gain or loss, no victory or defeat, no famine or plenty, was ever accidental or whimsical, since God was, either directly or indirectly, the first cause. He was the direct cause when he ordained a particular fate for a specific individual or nation and the indirect cause when a man or nation set his face against God and rejected the path of virtue. Psychological, physical and political misfortunes alike were commonly regarded as either punishments or penances for man's sins. Nowhere is this belief better typified than in the words of the last chronicler of the monastery of Peterborough. In the mid-twelfth century he wrote that for nineteen years, under the reign of King Stephen, the men of England were plagued by taxes, famine, poverty and pillage and thus they "suffered . . . for [their] sins."[11] Like famine and poverty, disease was inextricably intertwined with sin. God caused disease in a variety of ways.

He intervened directly by striking the sinful and sometimes the virtuous with unforeseen immediacy. One of the principal examples often cited in the Middle Ages is the episode of the ten plagues of Egypt found in Exodus. Here God proclaims himself the agent of misfortune and carries out his threats to punish all those who will not let his people sacrifice to him and bids Moses warn Pharaoh, "Behold my hand shall be upon thy fields: and a very grievous murrain upon thy horses and asses, and camels and oxen, and sheep" (9:3). Several verses later, God intensifies his punishments and extends them to men, saying, "for there shall be boils and swelling blains both in men and in beasts in the whole land of Egypt" (9:9). Later in Exodus, God himself slays the firstborn. In these instances, we see direct causation, first of symptoms of disease and later of death without apparent symptoms.

God might also cause disease in a somewhat more indirect manner through changes in the weather or changes in the arrangement of the stars. For example, in Exodus, the rain or hail and the locusts too destroy the crops, causing the diseases of famine. During the plague of the fourteenth century, those physicians and theologians who believed that hot, wet weather and bad winds caused the plague, knew that God was responsible for the wind and the rain. As the doctors of the first chapter noted, personality was predetermined and was consistent with the star under which and the season within which a mortal was born. Personality and humoral type predisposed a man to diseases of certain kinds. God disposed the star under which each man was born and thus predetermined both his humoral type and the consequent diseases to which he was subject.

God works indirectly through human agents, too. He may work through the Old Testament prophets, who represent just men, as he does in Deuteronomy when Moses expounds the laws and the commandments of the Lord to the Israelites. "May the Lord set the pestilence upon thee" (28:21). Here Moses, empowered by God, blesses those who keep all God's commandments with fruitfulness and prosperity, and curses all the disobedient with barrenness, famine and many other diseases of flesh and mind. The curse of the just man who is God's emissary carries the power of immediate and divine fulfillment. Thus, the wish is father to the deed, since the wish itself is implanted by God.

Last, God may work indirectly through either angels or demons. God may send angels to do his bidding and, in some instances, the angels, perceiving the wickedness of sinners, strike them with disease, as they do in the case of the sinners of Sodom, whom they blind. Numerous other cases of the use of angels as agents of disease in the service of divine vengeance appear persistently in medieval stories. Here the angels are usually disguised and the sinners do not recognize them because wickedness impairs their spiritual, hence their physical vision.

The evil and the virtuous alike were also prey to the devil and even to the pandemonium which might inflict a variety of diseases upon them by various means. The devil might simply enter into the body of a man, as Hilde-

gard of Bingen suggested, upsetting his humoral balance
and thereby bringing on disease. The devil might enter
into the mind of a man, thereby debilitating or destroying
the mind which controlled all other physical functions.
The devil might tempt a man to excesses leading to ill
health, either through sin or through physiological disorder caused by overindulgence. Last, the devil or one
of the devils might mount a direct assault against the liver
or the spleen or the eyes or indeed any and all physical
functions. These afflictions appear in the cases of the demoniac and the paralytic of the Gospels who are cured
by Jesus through a casting out of the devil. The old devils
were especially threatening in the Middle Ages. Well into
the Christian era, paganism survived either openly or in
various guises. The pagan pantheon of gods and demons
died hard and, although the church sought to kill the old
gods, it frequently found that this deicide could be effected most efficiently by assimilation and degradation.
Hence, Apollo became a demon and the old storm god of
the Germanic tribes, Herlikin, became a devilish leader of
riotous sinners. So, too, many old gods became specialized
devils for isolated diseases.

The agents whom God chose, like the diseases he in-
flicted, were consonant with the purposes the disease was
intended to serve. In the biblical tradition, which survived
in full strength throughout the Middle Ages, disease had
three principal functions. It was God's mode of punishment for sin, principally the sin of faithlessness; it was
God's way of testing a man's mettle, as in the case of Job,
who was afflicted with ulcers from head to foot so that
he cried out, "My bone hath cleaved to my skin and nothing but lips are left about my teeth" (19:20). In Job's
case, disease was also a purgation, for, suffering so on
earth, he was cleansed of the sins of this world and made
meet for the perfection of heaven. Disease was also an
instrument of warning to repent and, therefore, simultaneously a sign and symbol, an example to others of the

appearance of sin. Just as the eyes are called the mirror of
the soul, so, in the Middle Ages, the body was not infrequently a reflection of both the mind and the personality
or humor. Maculae on the flesh bespoke maculae on the
soul. Impurity of the soul was filth of the flesh. The ingenuity of justice in the ascription of medieval disease
was so highly refined that each disease was perfectly attuned to the measure of the man afflicted or, as Sophar
observed in the Book of Job, "according to the multitude
of his devices, so also shall he suffer" (20:18).

### Test

The martyr or saint is refined by temptation or agony,
and one of those agonies of the just man is disease. The
juster and more resilient the saint, the more terrible will
be the test, for sainthood is not easily attained. Every
medieval saint suffers in patterns consonant with the sufferings of Job and the temptation of Jesus. At each moment that the saint reaffirms his faith, new scourges are
applied until, at the last turn of the wrack, still clinging
to his faith, the saint passes from mortal agony to immortal bliss. For the disease which is perceived as test,
there is obviously no medical cure. Health will be restored
when the soul firmly establishes its virtuous domination
and triumph over the flesh. The medicine, if there is any,
is metaphorical and spiritual and must be administered
by the metaphorical physician, Jesus. Steadfast faith in
the face of suffering was the fee the diseased paid the
physician.

### Purgation

Disease as a purgation of sin is also medically incurable
and, if the reason for the disease were clearly understood,
no believing Christian would want to cure it, for the disease itself was the cure for eternal damnation, or a prom-
ise of salvation. Sometimes the chastened survived to
teach others the lesson which suffering had taught him

and sometimes he did not. When he received news that the plague was about to spread to his district, the Archbishop Zouche warned his flock in 1348 that some men might die because God chose to favor them, but others might die because they were especially dear to God. "For almighty God sometimes allows those whom he loves to be chastened so that their strength can be made complete by the outpouring of spiritual grace in their time of infirmity."[12] Though the man blessed by such chastening should not wish to cure his illness, mankind has always wanted a release from suffering and, to this end, various attempts to cure by various methods were tried. These attempts were justified by a lingering question. Was this agony God's reward or his punishment?

## Punishment

The predominant view of the cause of disease was that it was God's punishment for sins. This traditional concept did not originate in the Bible, for it has been common to many cultures. For example, Sophocles depicts the sufferings of the entire populace of Thebes, who have been afflicted with plague because of pride, patricide and incest of which their king, Oedipus, is unconsciously guilty. When the sinner becomes aware of his sin, he atones for it and his penance releases the populace from the torments they suffer. Disease here serves some of the same functions and is understood in many of the same ways that it is in Leviticus, where the leper is described as a man ritually unclean. This leper pollutes, not merely by contagion but by insidiously corrupting his neighbors who are exposed to impurity. In medieval literature leprosy is generally caused by pride of spirit and is often associated with the sin of lust.

Yet even the belief that sin lay at the root of disease did not preclude medical learning; clerics were not averse to the application of such therapies as diet, psychotherapy, leechcraft and chemotherapy. Some, like Arnold of Villanova, even warned against superstitious pursuits like collecting curative herbs by moonlight. Yet this same Arnold noted that another effective cure for disease was to cast a medal inscribed with a lamb and the words "Arhael tribus Judeii," and to hang this medal about the neck of the afflicted. The result is that ecclesiastics took advantage of both physiological and spiritual treatments, but prayer and penance were likely to be utmost in their minds. Providing that the disease could be ameliorated by human medicine the more physiologic treatments might work, but it never hurt to strike at the first cause of disease and this, most doctors agreed with the physicians of the soul, was always God. Just as modern physicians speak of treating "the whole man," so medieval practitioners sought to treat the whole man, and this no one could do without cleansing the soul. The influence of the church was always felt both in epidemiology and in the care of individual cases. The epitome of this sentiment is found in Ecclesiasticus (39:9,10), in which the sick man is urged "in thy sickness neglect not thyself, but pray to the lord, and he shall heal thee. Turn away from sin and order thy hands aright and cleanse thy heart from all offense." Here is the fiat for all Christians to persist in the pursuit of natural and physical cures but to put his trust chiefly in the help of God.

## MENTAL DISEASE

Insofar as insanity was a disease it did not differ from any other diseases in respect to etiology. Yet, as other critics have pointed out, it was among several diseases, leprosy and plague to be specific, which aroused the greatest terror and revulsion and sense of helplessness in medieval men as it does in modern men. Some of the medieval responses to the human mind and its dysfunction clarify medieval responses to insanity, but they do not entirely solve the mystery of the horror provoked by insanity. Further illumination can be sought in contemporary attitudes toward insanity which bear striking parallels to those of the medieval world.

First, medieval men, like men of the twentieth century, believed that what differentiated men from all other creatures, what defined their humanity, was that "reason" which, St. Augustine pointed out, God gave to man. Without his reason, man was a beast. Bestiality was the medieval metaphor for that most horrifying of all periods, the pagan, the unchristian state of man. A popular medieval figure who originated in the Celtic nature religions and survived even the Renaissance was the wild man. A half-human, half-ape creature, he lived in the woods, murdered men and beasts, ate their raw flesh and satisfied his lust by raping any woman who ventured into his domain. The embodiment of the medieval id, the wild man was an alternately attractive and repellent creature who satisfied his appetites without consequence, but who also served as a reminder of the pagan past with its forests and its nature religions, so terrifying to the civilized men of the Middle Ages. The most famous of all medieval wild men was the biblical prototype of the figure, Nebuchadnezzar.

In Daniel, chapter 4, Nebuchadnezzar "was driven away from among men, and did eat grass like an ox, and his body was wet with the dew of heaven: till his hairs grew like the feathers of eagles and his nails like birds' claws." The commentary he drew throughout the Middle Ages is voluminous and enlightening. He is seen as a type of the wild man, as a madman and as the devil.[13] The Bible tells us that Nebuchadnezzar was punished by this loss of his humanity because, when he became the mightiest of kings, he was overwhelmed by such pride that he forgot God. When he rejected human reason and followed the depraved instincts of beasts, he was transformed into a beast. Isidore of Seville called him "a type of the devil who led ensnared heretics into the captivity of error, that is he led the Church into Babylon and the ignorant into confusion."[14] Pierre Bersuire, a fourteenth-century commentator, tells us that Nebuchadnezzar lost his human form because he had the "wild and impious heart of a beast, full of cruelty and sin."[15] Medieval men who saw the constant threat of the devil in the ever-present attractions to the pagan rites of the past, summarized these temptations in the image of irrational bestiality. They feared its encroachment and spoke of it in the terms of St. Maximius, who had said that "the language of those is more serious and incurable who are deceived by the sweetness of delusions and are unhealthy in the guise of outward health. Are not all of those false and mad [falsa et insana] since they were made by God, when they change into sheep or beasts or into monsters of depravity?"[16]

The lesson is clear. The man who dresses in pagan skins, like the man who loses his reasonable piety, is seen as sick, mad and a beast. Man turned beast is the archsinner, the basest and most unnatural of all beings. He belongs nowhere and he is an outcast because he is insanely sinful and sinfully insane. Like the men of the Middle Ages, we call the flagrant madman "unnatural," "barely human," and we say that he has reverted, that he "acts like an animal." What makes him unnatural is, of course, especially repellent to the church. He is outside the community of men because he has lost his ability to know God. Tertullian said that "the mind cannot be separated from the soul, inasmuch as it is nothing more than the property or apparatus by which it knows . . ."[17] If knowing is a property of the soul, then the man who loses the instrument of knowledge, reason, has also lost his soul. A lost soul was damned and every medieval man knew this. Christian and Greek moral attitudes toward insanity intersect in the Greek maxim that "those whom the gods would destroy, they first drive mad."

Less philosophical and more immediate is a moral certainty which grows out of physiology, that the loss of the

logistic ability would end in the destruction of the body.
Bartholomew of England said that the spirit which "is
man's reasonable soul" is the "means by which the soul is
joined to the body; and without the service of such a
spirit, no act the soul may perfectly exercise in the body.
And, therefore, if these spirits be impaired, or let of their
working in any work, the accord of the body and soul
is dissolved, the reasonable spirit is let of all its work in
the Body. As it is seen in them that be amazed and mad
men and frantic and in others that oft lose use of reason."[18] Without reason, man may lose not only his immortal soul, but also the functions of his mortal flesh. It
is reason which maintained the balance of the humors,
established authority over the passions, controlled the
lower organs. Without reason, man lost the order that
binds flesh to will and limb to limb.

In the great scheme of ecclesiastical order, sin was the
villain. It might cause insanity or it might originate in
insanity, but the final result was a deviation from nature
and God's pattern. One sin led neatly into another and
the patterns of development were traced in poetry, drawings, carvings, which warned men that they must recognize the fatal conclusion to which initial sin would inevitably lead. In many medieval books we find drawings of
trees of sin. The root of all vices is usually pride, but pride
ramifies to wrath and wrath to despair. The Latin word
for despair is "tristitia," the same word which medieval
physicians were to use for the suffering experienced by
the humoral melancholic who lost his natural warmth.
Vincent of Beauvais defined tristitia as the ingoing of the
natural heat of the body. The spiritual symptom of melancholic humor was despair, the lack of faith in the mercy
of an infinitely kind God. Judas, the archetypal suicide,
was the prototype of the desperate sinner and his act was
considered the natural consummation of melancholia. The
taboo which touched both the madman and the suicide
also identified them with one another. It survives even

in the twentieth century, in which we, like medieval churchmen, consider madmen potential suicides and all suicides proven madmen. Progressive thinkers in the modern Catholic Church argue that it is permissible to bury suicides on church ground because the suicide is a man not responsible for his actions by reason of insanity.[19] The major difference, then, between the medieval and the modern response to insanity is that what the theologian of the Middle Ages called sin, we call sickness. Ironically, the doctrines of our humanistic era imply that modern man has perhaps even less free will than medieval philosophers accorded him.

None of these explanations of the horror of insanity is as prevalent or as frightening as the medieval fear of chaos or disorder. Perhaps the commonest and truest cliché about the Middle Ages is that it was a period obsessed with order. Despite the number of variations and innovations in medieval schemes of the universe, a prevailing sense of system and pattern is always discernible. There are charts of the hierarchy of vices and virtues, texts describing the order of physical and psychic functions, treatises on the ideal descent of political and ecclesiastical power. Legal documents defined the order and priority of financial and social duties. Even the books of rhetoric name the order and means by which a writer and speaker should describe a person. Order was essence of being or, as St. Thomas called it, God. For a number of reasons, the Middle Ages was neither the beginning nor the end of the "rage for order."

Order is attractive because it can be comprehended. Comprehension is power, the power to determine and change one's own life and society at large. Insanity was the manifestation of an always threatening disorder. Depictions of incipient insanity in medieval fiction compare the disorder of the mind to the disorder of the world. When a hero like Chrétien de Troyes' Yvain begins to go mad, we are told that "a storm rose up in his head." This

storm, so common an image of chaos, is turbulent, un-
manageable; it turns nature upside down, destroying men
and beasts and even the peace of a political state. Storms,
in the medieval world, whether they occur within the
mind or in the forest, recall the time before the golden
age of Christianity, the terrifying barbarism of the hea-
thens, even, by implication, the moment before the
creation.

Like the storm, insanity was unbridled passion, unpredictable, incomprehensible, dark and ungodly. It was the
emergence and the dominance of the forces forbidden
man. Freud was later to call these forces the id and to
bid them to return underground, where they belonged,
present but controlled like the Eumenides. Under the
reign of such powers no civilization could thrive and the
conscience of the church felt obligated to condemn them.
It concerned itself less with the names for disorderly creatures, like "wild man," from Celtic mythology, or "melancholic," from medical treatises, and chose instead to dwell
upon the moral terms which described man's fight against
evil or sin. So it was that the commonest names for madmen used by the church were "demoniac" and "fool."

Toward the demoniac, the church was openly hostile.
It dealt in him with its ancient enemy and gave no quar-
ter. Yet, with two types of eccentric or unusual behavior,
those of the fool and the mystic, the church was cautious
in its dealings. It felt obliged to determine whether folly
was a sin, a disease or a state of blessedness and, finally,
to decide whether the visionary was a true mystic or a
charlatan, deluded by the devil. In its definitions of the
origin and types of folly and of special visions of the gifted
seer, church philosophy is often at its subtle best. The
mystic and the fool both fell outside the usual categories
of the insane and yet they were, under special conditions,
treated as mad. The mystic was mad when his visions
were believed mere delusions, but visionary figures in the
Middle Ages are never described in medical terms. Their

talents as well as their flaws are metaphysical. The fool, on the other hand, is a figure which attracts the rigors of many medieval "sciences"—law, theology and medicine. What the fool and the mystic share as figures is their detachment or dissociation from the ordinary world and so they are often confused with one another. It is instructive to move from medical examinations of idiocy to metaphysical praise of divine simplicity.

There is, of course, a familiar medical meaning for the fool. The fool is a man deprived of natural wit. Isidore of Seville distinguishes between dementia, which is slow to develop and temporary in its effects, and amentia, which is congenital and permanent. Amentia is classified as one of the forms of folly and is synonymous with fatuity, both medically and, in the eyes of the church, morally. The condition of folly which we call idiocy was known as stultitia. Vincent of Beauvais, in his great encyclopedia of the thirteenth century, takes a medical as well as a moral view of this state. He first tells us that it is a privation of or a defect in wisdom. Then, citing an early church father, Lactantius, Vincent says that "stultitia is the absence of right and goodness in both deeds and words and is caused by ignorance."[20]

Toward this condition the church had two paradoxical attitudes which may, in fact, be reconciled by a clear understanding of the two major types of folly—natural and unnatural. Natural fools were born idiots who were socially treated as insane creatures suffering, not from a rejection of intelligence, but from an inherited absence of normal rational function. Often this form of retardation was salable. Fools were entertainers who might find employment by amusing the courtiers with their freakish pranks. But the aristocracy had refined tastes, refined often to the limits of perversity. Mastery of the court fool might amuse them as it did not the populace, who were as bewildered and often as frightened by the natural fool as we are today by the retardate. The natural fool was sometimes a ward of the king and a pet of the church. Those who exploited the profitable aspects of folly by pretending to be naturally stupid when they were actually what we might call "unnaturally clever," were known as unnatural or artificial fools. Last were the fools who were called so in the same sense that we casually refer to the excessive or the imprudent.

Toward natural fools the church attitudes are ambivalent. Generally fools are condemned, for folly is a sin and appears, as the art historian Emile Mâle pointed out, in carvings on the porches of such churches as Amiens and Notre Dame, and in many stained-glass windows, as the figure of the court fool carrying his overblown cudgel. Here the fool is intended to be contrasted to the wise or prudent or temperate man who knows God and uses his God-given wisdom to seek the measured path of virtue. The principal source and justification of the ecclesiastical condemnation of the fool is to be found in the medieval psalters which translate the fool of Psalm 52 as "insipiens," a scatterbrained or senseless man, who "said in his heart, 'there is no God.'" The psalmist tells us that God "will scatter the bones" of those who are so lacking in understanding ("intellectus"[21]) that "they fear what there is no cause to fear, yet do not tremble in the presence of God." John of Salisbury tells us in his twelfth-century *Policraticus* that ignorance of those things which should be known is culpable ignorance, and that anyone who is in the grip of that ignorance "joins the fools."[22]

That folly which is ignorance of God is condemned throughout the history of the church and it is often equated with that insanity which is a madness born of spiritual blindness. The terms "folly" and "insanity" here have no medical or physical sense at all. They are both used as moral pejoratives as they are still used today, but they evoke a horror far more immediate and more threatening in the Middle Ages than they do today, for medieval clerics, working out of a strong exegetical tradition of allegory, saw, in the court fools before them, physical types of a moral condition. The fool, with his irrational, manic act, his leaping, his distortions, his bizarre and impious humor, was often called a "natural" and seemed to remind the clerics of the dark forces within man, of a primitive folk tradition which still preserved that terrible rustic temptation—paganism. Thus, in many condemnations of folly, we find references to irrationality, bestiality, nature worship, impiety and insanity, confused and compounded with one another to produce that alloy which is monstrous sin against God and nature. Despite the warnings of the church, the alloy survived both within and without the cathedrals themselves. In the late Middle Ages many sermons decried the behavior of the young subdeacons who celebrated their feast on Circumcision Day, January first, not as a solemn day for prayer but as a *Festum Stultorum*, a feast of fools, during which they behaved like idiots and pagans, donning branches and animal skins and swinging from the very chandeliers of the church. They were called, by their more orthodox elders, "madmen," "animals," "fools" and "sinners," often all in the same sermon and always in one moral and spiritual breath.

In one of those complex reversals of attitude for which the ingenuity of medieval theologians is so famous, clerics throughout the Middle Ages occasionally praised a foolishness which they considered diametrically opposed to that internal quality of spiritual folly that St. Peter Chrysologus called a vanity or "that foolishness like a dementia."[23] This other foolishness was the naïveté praised in the Sermon on the Mount. They argued that the truly simple were pure in heart and that, because these simple natures were incapable of worldly sophistication, they were naturally attuned to God's wisdom. Their worldly incompetence was, in fact, the result of their harmony with the heavenly laws. As the medieval world began to wane, this view became increasingly popular. In the fourteenth century the Franciscans often referred to themselves as "mundi moriones," fools of the world, to emphasize the divine impracticality of the asceticism which made them voluntarily poor, the mendicants in a society of wealthier monastic orders.

Praise of worldly folly as divine simplicity was not to reach its zenith until the Renaissance, for the general moral view of folly during the Middle Ages was a negative one. Nevertheless, the concept of the fool as God's blessed simpleton long pre-existed the thirteenth century and we find early records of reverence for the moron in primitive societies which both predate and postdate the dissemination of Christianity. Yet, as the fourteenth century approaches, the praise of folly becomes somewhat louder and more frequent, almost as a harbinger and at once a cry against the approaching Renaissance humanism. Thus we find Chaucer, with an ear to the Bible and his tongue in his cheek, blessing the "lewed [foolish or simple] man," Langland telling us that simpletons who wander the countryside are "god's boyes" and "merry mouthed minstrals" and the church sometimes recommending charity and protection for these naïve children of God.

The mystic is a more problematic figure. One of the classic points of similarity between possession and certain positive spiritual states is the presence of knowledge and insight and experience in a person who had no access to these gifts by natural means. Fits of fear and trembling, the peculiar physical sensations of heat or light not available to ordinary mortals, could indicate commerce with the devil, but they could also reveal a supernatural unity with God. Just as we are prone to call the medieval demoniac a psychopath, so we are prone to call the medieval mystic a psychotic, out of touch with the real world. The debunking element in twentieth-century rationalism inclines to epilepsy as an explanation for Jesus' moments of mystical communication with God. Ironically, medieval theologians, although they expressed no doubts about the divinity of Jesus and the saints of the past, were perhaps even more concerned than we to determine whether the man or woman who felt God's warmth or heard heavenly voices was possessed, suffering from delusions, a mere religious profiteer, or a true mystic.

Margery Kempe, a fourteenth-century countrywoman of England, was prone to "fits," as she called them, during which she would moan and shriek in the very aisles of the church. She said that she was beginning to "madden for the love of God," but her skeptical and rather aggravated fellow parishioners deleted the phrase "for the love of God," except in those moments when they beseeched her silence. To most of them she was mad, to some she was a mystic truly given to the divine insight. The ability to know the truth of her visions was even more important to the medieval and modern believer than it is to the skeptic, for every believing Christian knows that the favorite and most ingenious trick of the devil is to deceive man in the guise of divinity.

Both the mystic and the demoniac are situated at the fringes of insanity, for, in the eyes of the medieval church, the mystic was divinely sane despite and even because of the fact that ordinary sinners considered him irrational. The demoniac was maddened because he was no longer a man. Not his own soul, but either the devil himself or a demon spoke through his mouth.

The medieval church took a moral view of madness which it sometimes condemned as vanity, deceit, ungodliness. It is that madness which St. Augustine purportedly described in the life of St. Monica attributed to him when he reviled himself for his "mad pranks" and for having followed men who were "blind with ugly madness of the false felicities of the earth." Though he recovered the "health of his body," St. Augustine cried, he remained "mad in sacrilegious soul."[24] For this madness the church of the Middle Ages had as little mercy as it had for the devil dwelling within the demoniac, for this was the madness born of earthly obsessions and immediate material satisfactions. For the mendicant madman the institution of the church prescribed charity since the creature was sick, albeit sin-sick. Yet, since all sickness was sin and Christ provided the example par excellence of love and sacrifice for the sinning man, the church often felt, officially at least, that it could do no less.

The parallels between medieval church attitudes toward insanity and our own do provide us with a greater understanding of the similarities between our age and the Middle Ages. We, like the medieval moralist, pity the poor demented but shun without remorse the criminally insane. We, like the theologian of the Middle Ages, see in many of the more violent forms of insanity a duality which R. D. Laing calls the "divided self." The chief difference lies, perhaps, in our concept of the origin of insanity. The earliest theologians and philosophers have noted, as LHermitte and Oesterreich pointed out, the complexity of the human soul. Medieval physicians noted the coexistence of the sensitive and appetitive forces within the human mind. They agonized over the tendency of the necessary lower impulses to gain domination over the higher. In periods of belief "in the omnipresence of diabolic forces, they have attributed these triumphs of the flesh over the spirit to diabolic powers. The duality which the exorcist sees in the possessed comes from without. A demon enters into a man, eradicating the former self and substituting his own will. The peculiar voices and dark impulses which emerge come from an exterior force.

In the modern psychoanalytic view, man's duality is inherent. Not only the lower forces but even the devils lie within man. The original force of the psyche, according to the Freudian view, is desire, lust for the physical, insistence upon gratification—the id, the old villain of original sin. The superego, the modern conscience, is ingrained not by God but by man.

In the constitution of the medieval psyche, there was

no conscience, there was only reason which impelled a man toward godliness and virtue. Modern psychology countenances the normality of conflicts within the individual. Medieval psychology views the conflict as a battle between erring flesh and virtuous reason. Hence, for post-Freudian man, the voices which speak out of the dark reaches of his soul represent hidden or repressed portions of the self. The voice of virtue which says no to the thunder of desire is our own conscience, which orders and educates our own libido. The voice of virtue in the medieval man was the spark of divinity, the reasonable soul, which struggled against the promptings of the devil. We have come to believe that, instead of being possessed by the devil, we possess the devil who lives within us from the moments of our earliest desires. Original sin is still with us, but it has been transmuted into original guilt for sins committed not by our forebears but by our biological natures. If these urges of the id and these needs of the ego cannot live in harmony with the superego, Freud finds a splitting, a duality which is the nature of the schizophrenic.

The last holdouts against the influence of Freud, like LHermitte, object bitterly to the fact that "not even the devil has escaped the clutches of the psychoanalyst."[25] A survivor of the orthodoxy of the medieval church, the exorcist, like the believer in possession, decries the vanity of searching for the secrets of possession in the realms of psychoanalytic theory. LHermitte and the demonologists of the church may well be prophetic in their acceptance of the ancient forms of forces beyond our knowledge. As E. R. Dodds, author of *The Greeks and the Irrational*, pointed out, nearly every period of extreme rationalism was followed by a return to the most ancient beliefs in a devil-beset world. Men could not bear the responsibility of the guilt inherent in that system of skeptical humanism which traced the origins and the consequences of every act to man alone.

In our own age we are witnessing a recrudescence of popular belief in supernatural forces which control our lives. We play tarot, we consult the ancient Chinese *Book of Changes,* we read with pleasure and half belief of satanic rites, and we wonder about diabolical forces which contain political systems. We even conduct experiments to prove that thought can direct the lives of plants and animals and we have begun to wonder just what the word "sane" means in an "insane world." In the conclusion of his influential book on possession, T. K. Oesterreich wrote that our knowledge of parapsychic phenomena is too limited to enable us to determine whether or not the ancient documents about prophecy and the ability to know and foresee the future, to sense devils and to deal with them, are true or false. "We must defer an answer to these questions until we know more of parapsychic phenomena, their frequency and conditions of origin. The purely negative reply which so greatly facilitated for rationalism the historical criticism of all these accounts is no longer possible."[26] Oesterreich wrote these words in 1921 and they ring even more soundly today.

We have learned bitterly to be skeptical of our skepticism. We seek new religions and new cults which were first born in ancient China and India and the Christian Middle Ages. The final irony today is that, as in the Middle Ages, the uneducated are more skeptical of the powers of the new mysticism than are the educated. It is the sophisticates today who look for internal harmony in external forces and who question the meaning and definition of sanity. In the new age of many faiths which grows out of an age of faithlessness, the civilized explorers are those who want to discover the islands of the irrational and to penetrate their secrets. The fine line between the spiritually gifted and the psychically unbalanced was perhaps best summarized by the mythographer Joseph Campbell, who noted in a lecture in 1973 that he had concluded in a discussion with a group of psychoanalysts that "the mystic and the lunatic both enter the same dark waters" and that the difference between them was that in these waters "the lunatic drowns, but the mystic swims with delight."

# CHAPTER III

## THOSE WHO DO NOT CONSENT
*The Insane and Medieval Law*

> Those who do not consent have not guilt . . .
>
> —GRATIAN

The medical treatises of the Middle Ages indicate the state of theoretical physiology and psychology, including the ancient traditions adapted to medieval medical teaching and practice. The religious commentaries embody the moral and philosophical doctrines of reason which, formalized by ecclesiastical acceptance, achieved the status of orthodoxy. Both the scientific and the ecclesiastical literature indicate what society was supposed to think about insanity. Neither tells later generations how the insane were officially received and treated by society at large. The law, however, has always been the executive agency of ideal social behavior and its actual enforcement. Of course, laws are not always enforced but they do reveal the attitudes and courses of action considered righteous and just and, at least occasionally, realized. The laws also manifest the attitudes considered unjust and abusive.

To investigate the laws of a society is to demonstrate the formalized conjunction of internal feeling and external action, to articulate the presumptions about individual relations to the larger social structure. The very existence of a law confirms a felt need to prevent either foreseen or observed social abuse. In medieval and ancient society, numerous laws were devoted to the rights and forfeitures of the insane, a fact which proves that insanity was a state familiar and frequent enough to require specific provisions for care, treatment and responsibility. There was no "law of the insane," per se, in the ancient or medieval era, but law governing the treatment of the criminally insane appears under the heading of criminal law, laws governing the marriage and testamentary powers of the insane appear in family or marital law and testamentary law respectively, and so forth. Each category of laws must be separately examined and many indicate the vast distances between ideal and actual treatment of the insane. By indirection, many of these same laws manifest a farsighted and complex concern that justice and mercy be meted out to those who could be so easily deprived of all rights and property.

The desire to be evenhanded demanded that the interests of lawyers should lie not in the diagnosis or cure of the disease, nor in the moral lessons to be drawn from it. In cases of madness, the lawyers of the Middle Ages saw their task as identical to that in cases of criminal behavior. First, the law had to define insanity and then to establish its existence in a particular case. From these two acts followed the determination of the status of the mad and, finally, of the rights which should be accorded to or denied them. All the major European legal systems which provided for the mad defined insanity in functional rather than in diagnostic terms. The law cared less whether a man was manic or melancholic than whether he was capable of responsibility for his behavior or, to be more precise, capable of acting within the law. Knowledge of the severity and duration of his state was essential to a just determination of the protection or punishment he should receive, and, in these two areas, law was dependent upon medical information. Just how the lawyers and judges obtained this medical information is not clarified in the legal documents of the period, but the first great forensic psychiatrist, Paolo Zacchia (1584–1659), clearly implied that experts in psychiatry were not always consulted when he recommended medical testimony as an ideal for his day and suggested that it was only a some-time practice of earlier periods in legal history.[1]

The legal history of insanity is so long and complicated that a brief aside is essential to an understanding of the origin and development of the laws with which medieval judges were dealing. The high point of European law in the Middle Ages is, like the high point of medicine and literature, the twelfth century. Again, as in the teaching and writing of medical doctrine, a single school surpassed all others in the production and dissemination of legal materials. This was Bologna, which succeeded Pavia, as the greatest law school of medieval Europe. The two greatest systems of medieval law, Roman law, called "civil law" (but encompassing also criminal law), and canon law, were explicated, modified and codified. The influence of barbaric, pre-Roman law, known as customal law, was often felt in the later commentaries on the ancient and traditional laws of Rome.

The most cursory glance at the history of law in what we today call "Europe" and "Britain" shows the progress of the gradual conquest by Roman law of the old, un-written customal laws of the barbaric tribes. Customal laws were, just as the name suggests, the body of un-written custom practiced with the regularity and force of law. There were as many customal laws as there were barbaric tribes. As the Romans conquered the various ter-ritories of the Alemanni, the Visigoths, the Ostrogoths, and others, each tribe began to feel something of the flavor, though usually not the wholesale imposition, of Roman law. However, the barbaric customs survived and were first codified after the fall of Rome and the establish-ment of kingships among the tribes-becoming-nations. By the fifth century, the Germanic Visigoths, who gained con-trol of a portion of Gaul and Spain, were writing their customs in Latin and showing the influence of the laws of Rome. Furthermore, the Roman religion, Christianity, ad-

hered to the Roman laws, so that, for example, any ordained clergy among the Merovingian Franks adopted
Roman law. As direct government of empire receded from
the barbaric territories, they turned increasingly to the
things of Rome and, if the law of Rome did not come to
them directly through the adaptation of Roman codes by
their kings, it came to them indirectly through the adaptation of Christianity.

This conversion to Roman law was not performed in an
instant and strange laws were practiced in the name of
Rome by its new subjects. A number of nations retained
their old laws and the most familiar of these to historians
of Europe is England. English common law grew out of
an attempt to reconcile the Anglo-Saxon and Norman
laws with the king's law. Starting with the reign of
Henry I in the early twelfth century, itinerant judges trav-
eled over the English countryside dispensing the king's
justice and, by the reign of Henry II in 1166, justices from
the exchequer, or royal household officials, toured the
shires to rule in cases and levy taxes. The collected decisions of these justices formed a body of precedent which
was the foundation of English common law. Yet, independent as the English considered themselves of the more
widespread legal systems of continental Europe, they were
inevitably influenced by Roman law through the agency
of the church. Church law was grafted onto the civil laws
of Ireland too and, through the influence of the church,
the laws of Rome were incorporated, to however small a
degree, in even the most independent of the medieval
"nations."

This universally influential church law, called "canon
law," was merely the body of laws which the church had
canonized. Its cornerstone was the *Corpus iuris civilis* of
Roman law, but it included decrees of church councils,
special letters on church issues written by popes or arch-
bishops, church rules, penitential pronouncements and a
score of other types of authoritative church pronounce-

ments on doctrine, policy and administration. Not until 1141 was this diffuse information collected, organized and elaborated upon in a single work. This was the *Decretum*, a compendium of decrees written by popes and councils and synods, then compiled and commented upon by Gratian, a monk who taught law at Bologna. His massive work surpassed in its comprehensiveness all earlier collections of canons and became the core of church law. Canon law did not end with the *Decretum*, however. Since the papacy was considered the source of all living church law, lower ecclesiastical courts appealed their problematic cases to the papacy. The popes and the papal curia answered these appeals with letters called "decretals," which also had the force of law. In this way, canon law continued to grow until, in 1234, Pope Gregory IX found necessary and useful the production of another classified compilation of these additional laws, which he called *The Decretals*. These two works, the *Decretum* of Gratian and the *Decretals* of Gregory IX formed the heart of medieval canon law, which Gratian's successors called the "new law" and we call the "corpus iuris canonici," the body of canon law.

Canon law has continued to grow since that time. There have been further collections of decretals, further decrees by popes, councils and synods, and, from Bologna, an inherited tradition of glosses (interpretative explanations) and "summae" (summaries) which flourished in the great encyclopedia-writing age of the thirteenth century. Canon law has undergone vast revisions and reconsiderations. In the early twentieth century a new body of canon law, called the "Code," was completely substituted for the old laws which grew out of the *Decretum* and various decretals and summae, including St. Thomas' summary of law. During the period after Gratian, canon law was called the "ius novum," to distinguish it from the old law, or "ius antiquum," which was the Roman law from which it grew. Canon law had jurisdiction over all matters which were the exclusive province of the church. These included the affairs of the clergy, cases involving church property and crimes against the church or the clergy. The jurisdiction over all clerical matters and all sacraments belonged to the church and the chief weapon which the canon lawyers wielded was perhaps the most deadly of all in medieval society—excommunication. Canon law held sway over a larger number of people and nations than any other single law of the Middle Ages, for Roman law was conceived of as a rule created by man, whereas canon law often had the cast of divinity and was generally considered closest to the "ius naturale," or natural law, the operation of God's will on earth.

When a case upon which no canon existed arose, the church turned to the source of its law, Roman law, so that any provisions neglected or unformulated by the church were already supplied by the earlier tradition. There is an old saying that the canons were worth nothing without the laws and the laws were worth little without the canons.[2] Those laws without which the canons could not have existed were the laws of the *Digest* (also called the *Pandects*) and the *Code*, a series of excerpts from classical authors and imperial enactments, compiled by Justinian in the sixth century. Roman law had, of course, been practiced by Roman rulers since the foundation of the empire, but the first important codification was the law of the Twelve Tables (c. 450 B.C.), a primitive law which was expanded over the course of the following several centuries. The classical period of Rome is generally considered the most fruitful in the development of Roman law, and the major surviving legal compilation of that period is the *Institutes of Gaius* (c. 150 A.D.).

The finest production of the law was not gathered into one major source until Justinian's books offered the lawyer and student an encyclopedia of the laws and works of all the greatest legislators. Both the *Digest* and the *Code* are divided into twelve books. The *Digest* was a compilation of civil law. The *Code*, only a second updated version of which still survives, was more varied. The major areas of jurisdiction included in its books were ecclesiastical law, private law (to which seven books are devoted), criminal law and administrative law.[3] Our modern concept of Roman law is formed by exposure to these works and several minor codices, the most famous of which is the *Codex Theodosianus*. But these works, since they were historical compilations, included traces of the ancient laws they were attempting to modernize for the sixth century.

While the canonists were teaching and compiling law at Bologna, they were in constant communication with the Roman lawyers there. Roman law had not been known north of Italy, except by a few literate (i.e., Latin-speaking) intellectuals, until the end of the eleventh century, when the manuscripts of the *Code* were transferred from the law school at Pavia, through Ravenna and Rome, to Bologna. From this time forth, the lawyers began to produce glosses, commentaries upon the original corpus of the law, which discussed, enlarged and altered the ancient laws to suit modern needs and systems. The first major gloss was produced at Bologna by a twelfth-century Tuscan, Irnerius. The most important of the glosses was that completed by Accursius in the mid-thirteenth century. It came to be considered standard throughout medieval Europe and was the major instrument of communication of the Justinian corpus. Slightly later, a school of commentators upon the law adjusted and expanded the "ius antiquum" to attune it more finely to new forms of government, customal law and canon law. The most famous and influential of these commentators was Bartolus of Sassoferrato (1314–57). Bologna, that hive of legal activity, was to both Roman and canon law of the Middle Ages what Salerno was to medieval medicine.

In the development of Roman law and in that part of the law adopted or created by the church, lies the history of the official status of the insane in medieval society. What becomes apparent in the change of emphasis which appears in canon law is an increasing interest in the technicalities of disease in general and of psychiatry in particular. Despite the fact that the Roman lawyers could have consulted the works of Hippocrates or the expertise of Galen and Aretaeus, in order to confirm a case of insanity, there is no direct evidence that they did so.[4] The earliest Roman laws which recognized the existence of insanity were devoted principally to the custody of property. The first of these is in the Twelve Tables, in which Law Seven states that "when no guardian has been appointed for an insane person, or a spendthrift, his nearest agnates [closest male relatives on the father's side of the family], or if there are none, his other relatives, must take charge of his property."[5] This laconic statement provides a great deal of information about the insane and Roman society. First, it informs us that the Romans had a system of guardianship which was either legally or familially organized. Second, it reveals a principal concern with responsibility for property, indicated by the fact that the mad and the spendthrifts are considered a class of legally irresponsible people whose irrationality was indicated by their inability to administer property in a judicious manner. Last, it tells us that those considered insane were maniacs because the Latin word for insane person here, as in most of Roman law, is "furiosus," a raving maniac.

This word "furiosus" is repeated in the next major law of the insane, a provision in the *Institutes of Gaius*. "An insane person cannot contract any business whatever, because he does not understand what he is doing."[6] This law repeats both the definition of the madman as maniac and the legal or, as it is called, "juridical" incapacity of the madman. It is a law which embodies the sense of all succeeding laws of Rome, for it declares a madman a nonperson in the eyes of the judicial system. It excludes him from all legal acts and all legal responsibility for acts he commits while mad. Considered in tandem, these two laws clarify the chief concerns of the Roman lawyers for the insane. With one hand, the laws of Rome gave protection to the insane and their properties; with the other, they took from the insane the right to any legitimate action. This balance between privilege and deprivation was characteristic of all Roman laws toward the insane in all areas of legal jurisdiction. A clearer illustration of the balance between privilege and forfeiture and of the social attitudes incorporated in the law appears in higher relief in the hypothetical case study of a Roman family.

Propertius, a Roman official, and his wife, Julia, had two children, a daughter, Fabula, and an older son, Titus. When Titus reached the age of manhood, his behavior became erratic. He did not seem to concentrate on what was being said. He had unpredictable rages and tantrums and he spoke to himself loudly and often. One day his mother, Julia, asked him to meet his father at the Forum and deliver a message. Titus lifted a heavy vase standing next to his mother and smashed it over her head, killing her instantly. Propertius returned home to find his wife dead and his son ranting. He sent Titus before the magistrates and, after examining the case, they concluded that he was insane. The judge ruled that Titus' father was to act as his curator, to administer all his affairs and supervise his care.

The judge was putting into legal effect the old Roman laws of guardianship, designed to protect both people and property. The system of guardianship grew increasingly elaborate with the declining power of the family or clan and the observation of corruption among appointed guardians, but it remained, throughout Roman law, the most important means of the social supervision of helpless people. Among the helpless were any child of prepuberty age and any woman of any age. Both of these had, from birth, a guardian called a "tutor." This tutor was usually the father because the power and supervisory authority of the father, called "patria potestas," over his sons was absolute until they reached maturity and over his daughters perpetually, since a woman was not supposed to be gifted with the strength, reason or logic to make legally binding decisions. When the child reached majority, guardianship remained in force in those cases in which it was needed, among which were counted "the case" of being a woman, the case of the spendthrift or the case of the legally insane or retarded. The title of the guardianship was then changed from "guardian" or "tutor" to "curator."[7] Sometimes the father or the earlier-appointed tutor remained, now in the position of guardian. Sometimes when, in adulthood, guardianship was no longer in force, new needs for a guardian arose. This need was apparent in cases of insanity which began in adulthood. In such instances either the father or the nearest male relative on the father's side (the agnate) became the curator, but the magistrates did have final authority to appoint any curator they saw fit; thus they could supersede the will of the family. Sometimes when a father who was the curator died or became incapacitated, necessity demanded his replacement by the agnate or another guardian appointed by the magistrate.

There were three major types of curatorship. A "curator testamentarius" was appointed by will; a "curator legitimus" was the agnate; the "curator dativus" was appointed by a magistrate. Although curatorship remained largely a matter of private and family law, increasing numbers of curators appointed by the praetor (an official who was subconsul or governor) appear as the family structure becomes more decentralized and the government increasingly diffuse after the fall of the empire in the fifth century. In cases of insanity, the lawgiver Ulpian had declared that the praetor should appoint a curator for anyone at the age of puberty (which was the age of juridical capacity) who was "not capable of transacting his own business."[8]

If a tutor had been appointed for a minor or a woman and the said person became insane, the tutor usually assumed the role of curator. If a curator for a madman was appointed, he remained guardian of the madman even after his recovery to sanity. The latter procedure was enforced so that endless curatorships need not be re-created in case of relapses into insanity, but the curator ceased to function during the so-called lucid intervals or remissions of the disease. During these periods the madman could act for himself without recourse to his curator.

The law protected not only children and husbands but the heads of the family. In Justinian's *Code*, a daughter is advised that, since her father is now insane, she should "petition to have curators appointed for him, by means of whom, if any business transacted should be revoked after proper examination, matters may be restored to their former condition."[9] In all cases of insanity, the function of the curator was carefully defined by the law of the *Digest*. "Not only the estate, but also the person and the safety of one who is insane, must be protected by the advice and exertions of his curator."[10]

The potential for curatorial abuse was both observed and foreseen by the Roman legislators. Guardians were once able to profit from their responsibilities by skimming off the cream of the income of their wards. To prevent such corruption and to protect the charge of the curator, the law stipulated that "the praetor must be careful not to appoint a curator rashly and without the most thorough investigation of the case." Curators were forbidden to take profit or accept monies for their administrative duties unless such acts were profitable to the interests of their charges. A curator was forbidden to alienate the property of the insane, to transfer any property including chattels, unless such an act benefited the insane person and that benefit was proved by a court investigation before the transfer. The pledge of a curator was valid only if the "benefit of the [insane] person required it."[11]

Titus would receive no punishment, but he would be chained. The statute to which the judge referred for his final decision arose from an old precedent in the case of one Aelius Perscus, who, while mad, had also killed his mother.

If it is positively ascertained by you that Aelius Perscus is to such a degree insane that, through his constant alienation of mind, he is void of all understanding, and no suspicion exists that he was pretending insanity when he killed his mother, you can disregard the manner of his punishment, since he has already been sufficiently punished by his insanity; still, he should be placed under careful restraint, and if you think proper, even be placed in chains; as this has reference not so much to his punishment as to his own protection and the safety of his neighbors. If, however, as often happens, he has intervals of sounder mind, you must diligently inquire whether he did not commit the crime during one of these periods, so that no indulgence should be given to his affliction; and, if you find that this is the case, please notify us, that We may determine whether he should be punished in proportion to the enormity of his offense, if he committed it at a time when he seemed to know what he was doing.[12]

Propertius was counseled not to berate or blame his son because "an insane person, as well as an infant, is legally incapable of malicious intent and the power to insult, and therefore the action for injuries cannot be brought against them."[13] Titus was, like all the insane, considered an infant, for neither infants nor the insane could injure anyone in a legal sense. Intention was at the root of legal injury and reason was essential in intent. Once the act had been committed, however, society had to be protected from the madman and the madman had to be shielded from himself. This was the rationale for placing him under physical and legal restraint. The criteria for determining his insanity were his lack of contact with social reality (i.e., degree of estrangement or social alienation) and his inability to intend or injure. Both arose from his more generalized inability to know what he was doing. Punishment was deferred or forbidden because insanity was considered itself a punishment—a concept derived from the ancient beliefs on godly vengeance.

Since Titus was to be guarded and chained during his madness, Propertius asked to know whether this decision would remain in force during his son's entire life. The *Code* of Justinian provided a medically oriented answer.

It sometimes happens that the affliction of insane men remains continuous and with others the attacks of disease are suspended and lucid intervals occur, and in this latter instance a great difference exists, for some of the lucid intervals are short, and others are of long duration. In former times, the question arose whether the authority of the curator continued to exist during lucid intervals of insanity, when it temporarily ceased, and when the disease returned, it was restored. Hence We, desiring to decide this doubtful point, do hereby decree that, as when insane persons of this kind recover their senses, it is uncertain and impossible to determine whether this will endure for a long time or for a short period, and as the parties in question frequently remain on the borderline of insanity and health, and after they continue for a considerable time in this condition, the lunacy seems in some cases to be removed, We decree that the appointment of a curator shall not be considered as ended, but to exist as long as the insane person lives, for generally a disease of this kind is incurable; and We also decree that, during their perfectly lucid intervals, the curator shall not exercise

his authority and that the demented person while
he is temporarily in possession of his senses, can
enter upon an estate, and do everything else which
sane men are competent to do.[14]

The legal prognosis for Titus was bleak, but his father's
only comfort rested in his certainty that his son would be
prevented from committing murder or suicide and from
squandering any property. Since there were no insane
asylums in Rome and no public facilities for treatment,
confinement or shelter of the insane, they were supervised in the private domain through the legal agency of
curatorship carried out through either the traditional
structure of kinship or the legal and governmental structure of praetorial appointment.

Because it was murder, Titus' case lay in the domain
of Roman criminal law and the criminally insane could
not be punished. As such, they were a privileged or special class of people incapable of doing harm ("incapax
doli") under the law, since they were incompetent to
know what harm was. Yet, just as they were protected
from punishment, so they were deprived of the right to
act legally for themselves. In criminal cases the insane who
were relieved of guilt were also deprived of freedom.
They could not give or receive, consent or dissent. They
had no will and could make no wills until and if they returned to "sound mind," however briefly. For any acts an
insane person committed after he had been placed in the
care of a curator, the curator was legally responsible.

Propertius' troubles were not over. One wonders if his
was R. D. Laing's schizophrenogenic family. Several years
after his wife had been murdered and his son had been
placed in his curatorial custody, Propertius concluded a
most advantageous marriage contract for his daughter,
Fabula. Her prospective husband, Fortunatus, received a
handsome dowry, and Fabula, informed of her father's
decision, seemed perfectly in accord with it. The couple

had not been married for more than three years when
Fabula too began to act as strange as her brother had
several years earlier. However, she did experience lucid
intervals and, although she shouted at servants and was
strangely alien toward her husband, she was not openly
violent. Fortunatus was a model of patience, reasoning,
as did the law, that although she might be insane, if a
spouse became insane but "had lucid intervals, or if the
affliction is perpetual but still endurable by those associated with the woman, then the marriage ought by no
means to be dissolved."[15] He knew also that "insanity
prevents the contraction of marriage, because consent is
necessary; but it does not annul it after it has been legally
contracted."

And where the party who is aware of this fact, and
of sound mind, gives notice of repudiation to the
other who is insane, he will, as we have stated, be
to blame for the dissolution of the marriage; for what
is so benevolent as for the husband or wife to share
in the accidental misfortunes of the other?[16]

Fortunatus knew that, despite her threats, Fabula, now
pronounced medically insane, could not renounce him, for
no insane spouse can repudiate his or her partner, "since
he or she is not in possession of her senses."[17] He continued to bear patiently with his wife's erratic behavior
and provided her with extra servants to attend her during
her bouts of rage and, throughout this course, was particularly careful to attend to her dowry, not only because
he was just and compassionate, but also because he knew
the law.

If, however, the woman is afflicted with the most
violent form of insanity and the husband, through
crafty motives, is unwilling to annul the marriage,
but treats the unfortunate condition of his wife with

scorn, and shows no sympathy for her, and it is perfectly evident that he does not give her proper care,
and makes a wrongful use of her dowry; then, either
the curator of the insane woman or her relatives have
the right to go into court in order to require the husband to support her, furnish her with provisions, provide her with medicine, and omit nothing which a
husband should do for his wife, according to the
amount of the dowry which he received.[18]

The dowry could even be sequestered so that a sufficient
portion of it could be used for the maintenance of the
wife and her slaves, and the marriage could remain in
force "dependent upon the recovery of the wife or the
death of either of the parties."[19]

Despite his patience, superb care and solicitude, Fortunatus observed that Fabula's condition was becoming
steadily worse. She began to strike her slaves and smash
the household goods. Her physician pronounced her dangerous and probably incurable. Fortunatus knew that only
two courses were open to him. He could repudiate his wife
under one set of conditions.

If, however, the insanity is so violent, ferocious, and
dangerous that no hope of recovery exists, and it
causes terror to the attendants; then, if the other
party desires to annul the marriage either on account
of cruelty which accompanies the insanity, or because
he has no children and is tempted by the desire of
having offspring, the said party, being of sound mind,
will be permitted to notify the other, who is insane,
of repudiation; so that the marriage may be dissolved
without reproach attaching to either; and neither
party will suffer damage.[20]

Fortunatus could also rid himself of this intolerable
burden if Fabula's father issued a notice of repudiation

on his daughter's behalf. As her guardian, he was empowered to do this, since someone had to act for a woman incapable of acting for herself. Again, the law both favored her and discriminated against her. A woman was supposed to tolerate her husband's insanity for five years before she repudiated him, but a husband could repudiate an insane wife after only three years.[21] On the other hand, the woman always had a guardian to protect her property.

Propertius decided to act on his daughter's behalf and to repudiate Fortunatus in order to recover Fabula's dowry, although he knew that he would have to spend most of it on his daughter's care. Had he deliberately deceived Fortunatus into believing that Fabula was sane at the time of the contract whereas she had actually been insane, he would have been guilty of acting without her consent and there might have been an easy annulment, but Fabula had been sane and had freely consented. Because all the requirements of marital agreements had been met and no deceit had been practiced, no annulment on grounds of illegality of the marriage was possible.

The Romans manifested concern for the welfare, especially of the mad wife, and for the property of the insane, and for the possible offspring of a marriage. It sought to protect the rights of children of the insane, by providing that:

> The children of a demented, as well as those of an insane person of both sexes can contract lawful marriage, and their dowries as well as the betrothal gifts must be furnished by the curator of their father and the amount of the same must be fixed in this Imperial City, by the most excellent Urban Prefect, and in the provinces by the illustrious Governor or the bishop of the diocese. This must be done according to the means of the person, in the presence of the demented or insane individual, and of those who are

of the highest rank in the family of all the parties concerned; so that, on this account, no damage may result to the property of the said insane or demented person . . .[22]

The *Digest* and the *Code* are both in accord that the daughters of lunatics and the idiots could marry, without the consent of an insane parent who was unable to give it. However, the law discriminated somewhat against male issue of idiots and the insane, suggesting either that the men passed on the genes for reason or that women were irrational in any case. The laws expressed some doubts about the ability of the son of an insane or demented parent to marry without first consulting the emperor. In all cases, the insane person who could not make contracts was assumed, by his inability to answer, to be tacitly consenting.

The aging Propertius spent the remainder of his days caring for his mad offspring, and when he was very old he prepared a will with some concern for the continued maintenance of his children. He, at least, was legally able to make a will because he was sane, the principal requisite for testamentary capacity. Yet Propertius, troubled by doubts, consulted the lawyers about a number of questions. Could his insane son inherit money? The lawyers answered that the son is entitled to his father's estate if he is the "proper heir of his parents and is his own master" but in any other case of "inheritance or succession, he could not accept an estate or obtain . . . possession of it while he was insane."[23] In such cases the madman's curator was granted authority over it. Propertius asked what the curator might do with his son's estate and was told that the curator was liable to administration of the estate for the benefit of his charge even if the curator was an agnate. "It is established that the property of an insane person cannot be dedicated to religious purposes by an agnate or any other curator of the former; for the

agnate of an insane person has not the absolute right to
alienate his property, but can only do so where the administration of his affairs demands it."[24] What would
happen to the care of his son and could he designate the
curator in his will? The curator designated by a dying
father for his daughter was considered legitimate and did
hold that position after the testator's death "provided that,
in this most flourishing city, he appears before the Prefect
of the same, and in a province before its governor in the
presence of the most pious bishop of the diocese and his
three coadjutors, and having placed his hands on the most
Holy Gospels, he declares that he will conduct all the
affairs of the said insane person lawfully and for his benefit, and that he will not omit anything which he may think
to be for his welfare, or permit anything to be done which
he believes will be to his disadvantage."[25] Only the decree of a governor could license the selling or encumber-
ment of the "rustic estates of wards or minors."

Last, in the hope that his son might one day return to
sanity, Propertius was concerned that he be able to administer his own legacy and to make a will himself. He
was told that "an insane person can make a will during a
lucid interval of his sanity." The same provisions applied
to the insane in testamentary law as those which applied
to the spendthrift. Because the insane were considered
incapable, they were also considered inculpable. Deprived
of the right to make a will, to dispose of legacies received,
to marry or to exercise authority in office, they were guar-
anteed special protection. Heavy penalties were imposed
upon families who neglected their insane relatives,
whether these relatives were children or parents. The
laws, for example, contained a special punishment for
children who fail to provide care and custody for an insane parent, asserting that such children "not only deserved to be disinherited, but also to suffer other penalties
prescribed by the law."[26]

So obvious are the benefits of a claim of insanity for

a responsible person that provision had to be made for
claims of inculpability on grounds of insanity. Ulpian had
noted that "many persons feign madness or insanity in
order that, by the appointment of a curator, they may
the more readily evade their civil obligations."[27] The
criminal laws stipulate close examination of the murderer
before sentencing him to a punishment which he may not
suffer if he is mad. In this evenhanded meting out of
protection and deprivation, we would expect to find
equality but, as usual, we find, instead, that certain
classes are privileged and that the wealthy or powerful
among the insane are entitled to more magnificent benefits than are the poor.

In cases of insanity the father or agnate may become
the guardian or the court may appoint one, "but if the
insane person is of noble birth, the senate must be called
together, and after investigation, a curator of the best
reputation and the highest integrity shall be appointed.
Where no such persons can be found, the appointment
shall be made under the sole direction of the Urban Prefect."[28] This law also protects the additional properties
of the wealthy, who, like the magistrates, had more to
lose. Ulpian said that "anyone who becomes insane is considered to retain the position and rank he previously held
and also his magistracy and authority; just as he retains
his property,"[29] but the law goes on to say that he cannot act on this authority until he regains his sanity.

His responsibility null because his ability to consent or
disagree was void, the madman at Roman law remained
in a position of stasis. He could not be denied his property, but he could be denied authority to dispose of it.
He could not repudiate a marital partner, any more than
he could take one. He could not be held responsible for a
crime, but he could not be left free to commit another.
If he were a wealthy or powerful madman, he had more
to lose through the ministrations of a corrupt curator and
additional provisions were made for his protection and

that of his property. Property was the principal concern of Roman laws governing the individual, and, for this reason, also of laws governing the care of the mad. Property defined citizenship and status, freedom and slavery. Yet, whether rich or poor, all madmen shared the legal privilege and burden of ignorance and legal incapacity.

In an edict which requires the presence of a person to complete a transaction, we are told that "an insane person occupies the same position as one who is absent."[30] He is further compared to a sleeping man, who cannot acquire possessions himself, for although he can touch them with his body, he has not the "disposition" to hold them. He is sometimes even juridically "dead." In order to be alive and responsible under the Roman law, a man or a woman had to be able to consent and dissent, an ability which could originate only in a lucid knowledge of what one was doing. Without this knowledge there could be no guilt, no intent or will, no capacity and, finally, no intelligence. These were the qualities in terms of which Roman law defined life and so the life of the irrational or insane man was in a suspension like sleep or absence.

Although Roman law never died, it grew at varying rates during different periods of history. During the twelfth century, it entered a new golden age when, especially at the school of Bologna, it inspired a burgeoning corpus of commentaries and additions. So brilliant were the teachers at Bologna that even papal decretals were sometimes addressed to this law school. There canon law came of age under the aegis of Gratian, who incorporated much of the old Roman law into his *Decretum*. The second or case section of the *Decretum* is highly indebted to both the *Digest* and the *Code*, although the question of each specific Roman source is still in process of investigation. Because canon law derived so often from Roman law, the most profitable way to investigate the force of the other most influential system of the Middle Ages is to compare the two systems of laws, for, as the lawyers of the church knew, a case not provided for by the canons was referred to Roman law.

Perhaps the major perceptible difference between Roman and canon law was the quality of philosophical inquiry peculiar to the laws of the church. In canon law, questions of reason, of authority and source and of the origins of law itself are examined in greater detail than they had been in the laws of Justinian. No doubt one of the major reasons for the philosophical cast of canon law lies in the fact that it rests, as does the tradition of patristic writing, upon the explanation of older texts. Furthermore, the second or case section of the *Decretum* requires commentary to explain the theory behind the case which has set a precedent. Statute law is inclined toward laconic statement, whereas precedent law is verbose and reflective. Last, canon law is theology in precept form; it is intended to be a subject for the speculation of priests and laymen. God's law, revealed in the Bible, always required explication so that mere mortals could understand the meaning of its revelation in actual events. Canon law attempted to reflect God's law, or "natural law" as it was called, but recognized that man's less than divinely perfect understanding required careful instruction. Since the church was concerned not only with temporal but also with divine justice, the substance of canon law differed in quality, if not always in point, from that of Roman law.

The movement of the church into the laws of insanity was really the legal invasion of the soul by way of the mind. The matters of sin, salvation, intent, compulsion and origin arise with great frequency in canon law. The distinctions between origin and type of insanity are finer than those in Roman law because the church was devoted to understanding the exact state of the soul, so closely related to the mind, and to the preservation of man's divine quality, his reason. In fact, the laws of the church, although they may deal with the same issues as do the laws of the Romans, are concerned less with crime than they are with sin. The canon lawyers, absorbed in spiritual or psychic questions, felt compelled to understand why an act was criminal and were not, therefore, satisfied with the mere decision that it was. They delved into the questions of motivation with minds sensitive to psychic function. St. Augustine had indicated the need for this dissection of the soul in the *City of God*.

We need not at present give a careful and copious exposition of the doctrine of scripture, the sum of Christian knowledge, regarding these passions. It subjects the mind itself to God, that He may rule and aid it, and the passions, again, to the mind, to moderate and bridle them and turn them to righteous uses. In our ethics, we do not so much inquire whether a pious soul is angry, as why he is angry; not whether he fears, but what he fears; not whether he is sad, but what is the cause of his sadness.[31]

Canon laws on insanity are preoccupied with two major issues: the salvation or damnation of the human soul; the protection of the "things of God," which included the sacraments, the property of the church, the priests, from the pollution of sin. The maxim of canon law might be: "Remember the church to keep it holy; remember the soul to keep it pure." The consequence of this dual concern was that canon law, like Roman law, both gave and took away. It offered the mad the mercy and protection of the church, but it also sheltered parishioners and their deserved sacraments from dangers attendant upon the abuse by the insane.

## THE TERMS AND THEIR DEFINITIONS

Before the guardians of church law could give or deprive they had to define insanity. The terms used to describe insanity in canon law were "amentia," "furor," "mens alienata" and "mente capti." Amentia meant general mental incapacity, usually or often originating at the earliest age of a man or woman and always considered permanent. Furor was rage or mania, and, like the extremes of passion, could abate. Those suffering from mens alienata were comparable to our schizophrenics and were out of touch with social reality or estranged. Those who suffered from mind "seized" ("mente capti") were often in the direct power of the devil or some external force which robbed them of the use of the mind. They were possessed by some other power and therefore not in control of themselves. Intimately related to people in seizure or captivity were those called the "compulsi" or the "impollenti." The first were driven, compulsives who were impelled by an external force. The second were powerless, both in terms of their juridical identities (i.e., legally powerless to act) and in terms of their dominion over their own minds. The term "irresistible impulse" is mentioned directly or by implication throughout canon law and is generally a motivation that exculpates anyone acting under it. Those in the power of an irresistible impulse are "unsound of mind" because they are the "nescientes," those who do not know what they are doing, a description borrowed from Roman law. They are also "incapax rationis," or "incapable of reason."

The terms "dementia," a generalized description of insanity, and "insania," another term denoting spiritual ill health, also appear in canon law. These technical terms were not always used with great precision. Roman law influenced canon law terminology, for the church adopted the general notion of "inability to know what one is doing," "inability to consent or dissent," "permanent insanity," "intermittent insanity with lucid intervals" and the consequent "unimputability" of crime or injury to the man with a mind so affected. Yet, because the church intervened where civil law did not, in the matters of the salvation or damnation of a soul, the determination of sin, and even in matters of healing through spiritual means, it became increasingly refined in its distinctions between types of insanity, or, to be more precise, degrees of insanity.

Although a number of canonists indicate that the medieval church was, like the Roman courts, uninterested in legal diagnoses of madness, we see in the fine classifications of St. Thomas that distinctions in type arise from a concern with duration. St. Thomas' four classes of the insane are: those who are insane from infancy without any lucid intervals; those insane from infancy who experience periods of lucidity; those who were once sane but have lost their reason; those who are mentally deficient but can, nevertheless, think of their salvation.[32] Certainly the last group suffers from retardation (amentia), whereas the first and third suffer from dementia and insania. The second group suffers from episodes of mania or melancholia.

## SACRAMENTS AND THE INSANE IN THE CHRISTIAN COMMUNITY

St. Thomas' interest in degrees and duration of capacity is motivated partially by his interest in the ability of a man to partake of the divine contract inherent in the acceptance of some of the sacraments. He, like all other canon lawyers, agreed that a man who cannot understand the sacraments cannot partake of the blessings and concomitant responsibilities these rites confer. The sacraments are not only wasted upon such a person, they are also profaned by him because he does not know what he is doing unless he is experiencing a lucid interval. Some sacraments are conferred upon the insane, but some require full knowledge and understanding. St. Thomas creates a clearer hierarchy of responsibilities, maintaining that lesser capacities are necessary for the participation in some sacraments, such as baptism, fuller capacities for participation in others, such as marriage and ordination.

The dispensing or withholding of sacraments was the

perquisite of church law. That they were offered or refused any Christian was a major factor not only in his social standing in the community of Christians in which he lived, but also in the community of eternity in which he believed. An unbaptized man or woman carried the stain of original sin into the next world; a man denied last rites died with the taint of sin upon him and might go to hell or purgatory. The man refused the eucharist was, ipso facto, denied the completion of other sacraments and the consummate Christian experience. Every sacrament carried with it status in a tightly knit spiritual and social milieu and, for this reason, the relation of the insane to the sacraments was central to their standing in the medieval world.

To the degree that consent or dissent was required of the participant in the rite, he might be denied the sacrament if he were incapable of consenting or dissenting. The earliest sacrament in the life of a man, baptism, was traditionally performed at an age when the issues of knowledge and consent were irrelevant. Because infant baptism was a sacrament for those who had not legally the use of reason, the sacrament could also be conferred upon the insane. Timothy, bishop of Alexandria (c. 385), and St. Augustine compared the mad to infants who could not exhibit intention in any spiritual matter. Nevertheless, they declared, the sacrament could confer benefits without requiring knowledge. Since the insane were, under both Roman and canon law, infants, they could receive baptism whether deranged from birth or mentally incapacitated at a later time. Since the insane were assumed to consent, they could always be baptized providing that they had not specified any unwillingness to undergo the rite. In cases of late baptism or baptism preceding death, the insane, like all sick men, were admitted to the sacrament providing that, before their illness or incapacity, they had expressed the willingness to do so. The rite of baptism offered to the insane a spiritual exemption similar to the legal exemption which insanity offered the mad. "After baptism, no sin can be charged, whether it be adult or child, unless he was capable of reason."[33]

Previous intention is the key to many of the laws governing the sacraments. Penance and the eucharist both required previous intention or simultaneous ability to understand, the principal ingredient of intention. Penance was readily accessible to the sick and the mentally deranged since they, like the infants discussed in baptismal laws, could derive spiritual benefits from the sacrament without understanding it, but there were severe penalties for administering penance to anyone not fully conscious if he had not, in a former state of full consciousness, expressed a desire for the sacrament. The priest who administered absolution following penance upon anyone irrational, who had not previously shown clear intention to take it, was subject to a sentence of excommunication for one year. The same requirement of previous intention applied to extreme unction.

The administration of the eucharist to the insane in danger of death was a tradition based upon the ruling of the Fourth Council of Carthage (c. 432). However, in Gratian's *Decretum*, we find that some special provisos apply to the eucharist. Obviously the body of Christ required rigorous protection from pollution or misuse. If a person were possessed, for example, or even for any other reason repelled by or incapable of holding the eucharist in his mouth, he was forbidden to take it. Those perpetually insane from birth were not permitted the eucharist. An insane person might abuse it or even let it fall to the ground and, in so doing, he was blaspheming against the Body of Christ. Not only did the insane man have to have once desired the eucharist, he had to be competent, even in his derangement, to treat it with proper reverence.

Two sacraments, marriage and ordination, were both understood as contracts. It could even be said that ordination was a form of marriage. Penance, baptism, extreme unction and confirmation were both offered and withheld because they marked a man's citizenship in the community of Christians and provided for his salvation. The eucharist was given or withheld because it conferred some of Christ's sacrificial divinity upon a man. All of these sacraments were exclusively contracts between man and God. Marriage and ordination, however, were contracts between both man and God and man and man.

## THE SACRAMENT OF MARRIAGE: COPULATION AND CONSENT

Under Roman law marriage was not considered a full contract, but under canon law it was a divine contract. We read in Roman law that "consent not cohabitation" constitutes a marriage. In canon law, too, consent was considered essential to a marriage. For the same reasons as those advanced by Roman law, the canon lawyers declared a marriage contracted without consent invalid. The insane were incapable of consent except during that famous "lucid interval." However, according to church law, a marriage, once contracted, became sacrosanct, so that no illness or misfortune was sufficient grounds for divorce. The church, once marriage was thoroughly established as a sacrament in the thirteenth century, was unshakably opposed to divorce, so much so that a second marriage, contracted after dissolution of a first, was considered adulterous. "Till death do us part," was the ecclesiastical dictum on marriage, "in sickness and in health, for better or for worse." This belief in the sacred indissolubility of marriage was a major contribution of canon law. Only in cases in which the partner of a marriage was mad at the time of contract and, therefore, legally incompetent to contract, could a marriage be nullified.

The second major contribution to the laws of marriage was the so-called "copula theory," propounded by a large school of lawyers toward the end of the twelfth century.

This theory, contradictory to the old Roman law of consent in marriage, proclaimed copulation, rather than consent, the irrevocable consummation of a marriage. One jurist, Rufinus (c. 1190), noted that partners could not be separated if the marriage was contracted and consummated before a party to it became insane. The principal effect of this school of thought was that it permitted annulment of any contracted marriage which had not been consummated. A number of cases in which the plaintiffs rushed to dissolve the marriage immediately after the vows prove the force and results of the theory, whose chief proponent in the twelfth century was the jurist Rolandus Bandinelli, later to become Pope Alexander III.[34]

## POLLUTION AND THE INSANE PRIEST

Ordination was, of course, the sacrament contract which carried the greatest temporal powers. The priest was a model to his flock, the pastor of their souls, the celebrant of the sacraments. Chaucer mentions the importance of a pastor when he proclaims that a "shiten shepherd" cannot have "clean sheep." The priest who was unfit debased his flock, endangered their souls and defiled the sacraments. Within many realms the clergy were exempt from temporal justice administered by the king's courts and justiciars, and, for this reason, they had to be governed by a legal body and a code of law empowered to act within and for the separate institution of ecclesiastical government.

Obviously no madman could be ordained. The reason offered by canon law was his incapability. He could not understand the contract he was making. The church was also opposed to the ordination of any man who had been mad or subject to epilepsy, on the grounds that the disease might recur. Gratian, quoting from the first epistle of Pope Gelasius to the universal bishops, said that some

people might be "enticed to burst forth to such an extent
that they may allow the sacred ministry to be controlled
by demons and the like after the passions have been ensnared. And if someone ordained for this work is attacked
with a peculiar necessity, who of the faithful is assured
of his own soundness when he foresees that the ministers
of human care themselves are shaken by so great a misfortune?"[35] He recommends that these men be removed
and declares that mental disability is worse than physical
disability. "Lastly, if the divine law by no means permitted those who were perhaps wounded in body or
crippled to come in contact with consecrated things, how
much more fitting it is that the dispensers of the heavenly
gifts should not be (what is worse) stricken in mind."[36]

Gratian proclaims that, although no one who has been
previously mad ought to be ordained, a man who became
mad after ordination should not be deprived of his orders
while mad, but must "abstain from . . . priestly office
unless by chance he happened to return to sanity."[37] The
legal justification for this canon is that the insane cannot
renounce office any more than they can accept it. Yet it
was the not so secret hope of the church that a mad priest
would, during a lucid interval, voluntarily, or even after
some persuasion, renounce his orders. During the course
of his insanity the priest was deprived of "the performance of sacred rites" because he "hinders the performance
of the sacrament."[38] "Those who are seized or those who
are epileptics may not serve at sacred altars."[39] Gratian
explains that no one who has been "seized by demons
and hurled down on the ground, or those who are carried
away by attacks of shaking, may dare to serve at the sacred altars or administer the divine sacrament by themselves while shaking, excepting those who, devoted to
mortification of their bodies, are shown to be knocked to
the ground without these kinds of sufferings; those who,
however, were away from their duties so long of their
own accord and were suspended in due order from their

position and who, for the space of one year, at the discretion of the bishop, may be found to be free from assault by demons."[40]

The intent of the law is clear here. The possessed abuses sacred objects and pollutes them by touch; the tremulous epileptic may dishonor or destroy the sacred objects of the church. In the course of listing the illnesses which prohibit a priest from performing sacred offices, Gratian distinguished, on the basis of far earlier documents, between "seizure by devils" and "attacks of vexation," thus confirming the fact that canon lawyers did distinguish, as did more philosophical theologians, between bodily illness, mental illness and possession.

## REASON, SIN, FREE WILL AND GUILT

These laws governing the admission to or exclusion from the sacraments are all examples of that portion of canon law based upon the standard Roman law criteria of knowledge and capacity to understand. Each of these laws was designed to protect the sacraments rather than to protect the parishioners. But the jurisdiction of the church over the souls of men extended far beyond the domain of the sacraments. In legislation which encompassed the official attitudes toward medicine, theology and psychology, the canon lawyers made extensive forays into the structure of the human mind. In its expeditions into the territory of the conscious and the unconscious mind, church law explored the relations between crime, sin, madness and illness which established the ecclesiastical rules of responsibility, culpability and even spiritual healing. To bare these interrelations, the canon lawyers studied the anatomy of the soul and the connections between this anatomy and the structure of a greater law which revealed the path to salvation.

The central element in the laws governing responsibility for soundness of mind or unsoundness of mind is St.

Augustine's doctrine of free will. Crime is understood here
as sin and sin is the chief concern of the forensic psychiatry of the medieval church. In a case entirely devoted
to the responsibility to be assigned to a priest who committed murder while mad, Gratian said that "those who
are out of their minds ought not to be blamed for [a
crime] or a sin."[41] His justification is entirely derived
from St. Augustine's statement that "it is . . . the will that
moves the soul either to avoid or to strive after something."[42] Gratian repeated St. Augustine's statement
that only the willing can be held responsible for their
actions. "This is the definition of sin, as we have said: sin
is the will clinging to or pursuing that which justice for-
bids, from which one should freely abstain, because in
truth it is such a great sin and not even because of punishment for sin."[43]

In his commentary upon the murder committed by the
mad priest, Gratian, saying that those who are mad should
not be blamed for their deeds since they have no free
will or free judgment, points out that St. Augustine had
said that "where there is no will, there can be no sin."
"Even if I sin through bad will, if it is not voluntary, in
no way can there be sin."[44] The mad, then, are those
who have no wills at all, and because they lack wills they
cannot freely consent or dissent. They live entirely under
the rod of compulsion. Madness is defined here in the old
Augustinian terms of loss or absence of will. It is defined
principally as "a weakness of the spirit."

> Likewise, the weakness of the spirit is twofold: one
> which is called a vice, by which the spirit is sep-
> arated from God, such as anger, hatred, and others
> of this kind: the other weakness of the spirit is that
> which, although it is not itself sin, causes sin and
> punishment, such as, forgetfulness and ignorance.
> Moreover, madness, although it is not sin, is, never-
> theless, a punishment for sin, as are fevers and all

other passions which we say are characteristic of the flesh. . . ."[45]

Although madness was often called "a weakness of nature," the church fathers and the canon lawyers held many men indirectly responsible for this weakness if it was caused by an initial sin. Under these conditions, a man was held responsible, not for deeds committed while insane, but for deeds and even thoughts executed and conceived before insanity. These sins could be punished by insanity. The church reasoned that insanity could not be the cause of sin, but it could be the result of sin. By indirection, a man was guilty of causing his own insanity, which the church considered a kind of slavery since it was predicated upon the absence of free will. "No one can be bound in the yoke of slavery unless he has first betrayed himself by sin."[46] This betrayal was inherent in the human condition, since "sin proceeds from" corruption of the spirit by reason of union with the flesh. Further, there is another weakness which properly is called of the flesh, because the flesh itself is affected and at length destroyed by that familiar medical problem, a disorder of the harmony of the elements of the humors.[47] Insanity here falls into the general class of disease. In this vein, the mad are compared to the drunk in the canon devoted to a murder committed under the compulsion of insanity. Lot is an illustration. He did not know that he was committing incest because he was robbed of his senses by drink, but he knew that he was drinking excessively. "Lot was not blamed for his incest but for his drunkenness."[48]

In a startling essay into the unconscious, canon law elaborated upon a man's responsibility for even his dreams. No man who had had erotic or otherwise sinful dreams was supposed to enter a church without first cleansing himself with water from a well (or tears), because his dreams were a form of pollution; canon law diagnosed the responsibility for dreams. "There is no sin when we are deluded by nocturnal images unwillingly; but there is sin at that time if, before we are deluded, we anticipate them with a favorable state of mind. Of course, images of excess which we carry on in real life often appear in the mind during sleep, but they are harmless if they occur without being sought after."[49] Gratian notes that we are guilty if "from the impure thoughts of one who is awake an illusion arises in his mind while asleep [for] it is clear that his soul is guilty. For it may be seen from what root that filth had proceeded because he considered it knowingly, he brought it about unaware."[50]

## PENANCE AND FREEDOM FROM GUILT

The church provided for the unimputability of the mad, but also demanded punishment for those who were not mad from birth, but who brought madness upon themselves through sin. Church law realized that all of life is a struggle between body and mind and body and soul. When the body triumphed the mind was defeated. The innocent mad cannot sin. "For they are not evil when the mind is not involved with crime nor are they bound by conscience. No one who is judicious will call poverty, obscurity, sickness, death evil; nor will he be counted among the log of the wicked."[51] Nevertheless, "those persevering in wickedness are excused through ignorance. But they will be brought to punishment whether it proceeds from weakness of the flesh or [like madness] weakness of nature."[52] "Therefore, whether sins occur due to the will or whether they occur due to weakness, they will always be liable to punishment."[53] The church which said it would not punish the insane seems to contradict itself here but, in fact, it does not. It punishes the sane alone, for an insane man must be returned to sanity before he does penance. Furthermore, he is to be understood as being punished not for what he did while insane, but for the causes which made him reach that point of insanity at which he could commit a crime. The punishment is seen as a form of teaching about sin, as a device for maintaining discipline within the church and as an instrument for cleansing the soul in preparation for death. So we are told that "one who killed someone while insane, regaining his mind, performs penance."[54] Gratian pointed out that the murderer cannot be punished for the crime he committed under the compulsion of madness but that he is responsible for that sinful condition which caused his madness. Often a lighter penance than that assigned to a perpetually sane criminal was assigned to an insane criminal who had regained his faculties.

The mad were insensible of punishment. Canon lawyers comforted themselves as we comfort ourselves when they proclaimed that the mad can neither give nor receive injury. "Those who are mad and those who are young are not capable of suffering pain. For those who are accustomed to suffer injury do not suffer."[55] One must know what he is doing, the canon lawyers asserted, to give injury or to feel it. In this way, canon law legitimatizes our eternal desire to believe that the mad cannot feel or that they do not know what others do to them. Yet, cold as this assertion may sound, it does not convey the entire spirit of the church attitudes toward the insane.


## THE SPECIAL MERCIES OF THE CHURCH

Just as it prohibited and punished, just as it denied and excluded, the church also offered special charity and mercy to the insane. They were treated with great solicitude in the matter of religious participation and the benefits of certain sacraments, largely on the basis of a law derived from the Council of Orange in 441. "Everything of piety is to be conferred upon the mad," proclaims the thirteenth canon of the council. Of course, the word for mad here is "amentibus," which means those mentally incapacitated from birth, and the things "of piety" do not include ordination and marriage. What sacraments they did include is not entirely clear except that baptism was obviously one of them and baptism eradicated all past guilt and all responsibility for subsequent sins committed before a return to reason or sanity. There is also evidence that the mad were admitted to mass, although one archivist believes that they were confined in an enclosed chamber behind the altar so that they could receive the benefits of the mass without harming their fellow congregants. The sinless mad could, of course, take the eucharist, providing that they were in a proper condition to hold it, and probably could receive last rites. Penance, for those perpetually mad who were baptized, was unnecessary, since they could not commit sins.

Madmen were also supposed to be offered special protection because they were helpless and like infants. For this reason, among others, they were not punished. Lighter penances after a return to sanity evolved not only because of the recognition that the mad were unaware, but also because the canon lawyers proclaimed that their principal concern was not punishment but teaching. Furthermore, the perpetually mad were never held responsible for their acts. "They are forgiven who sin unknowingly."[56] In a passage on Christian teaching, the author compared children to the insane and urged that they be taught despite their ignorance or resistance, saying, "It would be proper to heal them against their will, like the mentally deranged, except that to all belongs forbearance for such a sickness. For it is necessary, I believe, to teach, but not to punish the senseless."[57] Even in cases of suicide, mercy was accorded the insane suicide. The *Bigotian Penitential* says: "Anyone who kills himself while insane, prayers are said for him, and alms are given for his soul, if he was previously pious. If he has killed himself in despair or for any other cause, he must be left to the judgment of God, for men dare not offer their prayers for him—that is, a Mass—unless it be some other prayers, and almsgiving to the poor and miserable."[58] The mad suicide must have been virtuous before his madness or else he was guilty of the sin that caused his insanity and suicide. A previously virtuous or sinless insane suicide could have a Christian burial, but a sinful suicide could not.

Another major privilege of the insane was the right of sanctuary, even after the commission of a crime. Gratian noted that the will-less murderer should not be denied the opportunity for refuge. An earlier mandate of Theodosius II and Valentinian III, issued in 431, declared that "those fleeing for refuge and fearlessness and rashness and presumption and audacity and even insanity" should find sanctuary in the church so that they might not be denied "at least a single and final haven for wretched and helpless persons."[59] If, however, the mad refused to surrender their weapons and continued to act violently in the confines of their havens, the church seemed to beg off the right of sanctuary. But any mad or violent person who had laid down his arms in the protection of the church was defended from being dragged forth, and anyone who defied this right was subject to severe penalties.

Like the civil laws of Rome, the canon laws of the medieval world sought to provide for the future of the proven madman. Although the churchmen often referred to the rather complete Roman institution of guardianship, the church also expressed interest in furthering and perpetuating guardianship in an ecclesiastical jurisdiction. In 530, the authority of the church was introduced into the institution of guardianship when a canon declared that an appointed curator was to swear before a bishop and thirty other men on the Bible that he would "manage all things to the advantage of the insane."[60] In a canon from the Fourth Council of Toledo (c. 633), it was "decreed that clerics who, because of their age, stood in need of protection, should be placed under the guardianship of the

priests."[61] In this manner the church set precedents in
canon law, like those in Roman law, for the care of the
legally incompetent or those who needed special protection. On the other hand, Gennaro J. Sesto, a modern
canonist, emphasized the fact that the church encouraged
its officials to conduct their secular affairs through the
agency of others. The precedent for this condition, he
finds, was a passage in II Timothy 2:4. "No one serving
as Christ's soldier entangles himself in worldly affairs, that
he may please him whose support he has secured." Often
church officials were relieved of the responsibility of
guardianship since such a duty might involve them in
secular affairs, but we may assume that sometimes ecclesiastics could serve as guardians for a fellow churchman who had little relation to the things of this world.
In any case, the various means of appointing guardians
and curators underwent changes coincident with and dependent upon changes in governments and the structure
of civil appointments and duties. Yet the institution survived. Current authorities on guardianship have pointed
out that the old Roman manner of appointing guardians
remained in force until the establishment of the Napole-
onic Code, yet we know that minor variations appeared.[62]
For example, when, in the Middle Ages, the office of
praetor vanished, the judex selected guardians, or the
king appointed guardians in civil cases. What is important
is that guardianship remained the principal instrument of
social protection and supervision of the insane, and that
guardianship was, when recommended by the canon lawyers, executed largely by the instruments of Roman law
designed for this particular form of care. The greatest
care was cure.


## THE CHURCH AS A HEALER

When the church considered the sinful maladies which
caused insanity, it inclined toward areas which might be

considered the province of medicine. If madness were a
malady of the mind, and canon law translated mind into
soul just as it translated crime into sin, it was compelled
to consider cures which were spiritual. Priests, as agents
of God on earth, had curative powers which the more
secular physicians could not claim. Particularly in cases
of possession, but generally in all diseases (since, in the
eyes of the church, sin was at the root of disease), both
the madman and his ministering clergyman had to be protected against blasphemous or diabolic therapy. To this
end, Gratian, in the second part of his *Decretum*, cited
a law that said: "Incantations are not at all preferable
as remedies for the mental instability of men. Let the
priests remind the faithful people that they should recognize that magic arts and incantations cannot confer a
remedy for the mental instability of men; weak animals
cannot be cured either from lameness or from anything
deadly; but this is a snare and an ambush of the old enemy [the devil] who wickedly strives to deceive mankind.
And if anyone practices these things, let a cleric step
down, let a layman be anathematized."[63]

Obviously such a caveat indicated that all these forbidden methods were used. There are remarkable incon-
sistencies in the behavior and warnings of the church,
which decried magic yet practiced it. It is important to
remember, however, that some of the cures we consider
magical, they did not. Stones and herbs were supposed
by physicians, scientists and priests alike to have physical
rather than supernatural powers and so Gratian noted that
one is allowed to use herbs and stones providing that
their use is not accompanied by incantations. Gratian declares that these two therapeutic aids are of particular
benefit in "the restraining of demons." One could be mad,
church law recognized, without being possessed by the
devil and, in this case, one had to avoid, most scrupu-
lously, falling into a diabolic trap to which the helpless
might be particularly prey. If the madman was maddened

by possession he had nothing to fear from demonic cures, but the administering priest had much to fear.

## INSANITY AS A FIGURE OF SPEECH

In the largest sense, the church saw itself surrounded by insanity and feared it because it was an attack on individual souls, on Christian life and even upon the law itself. For the church, law, Christianity, salvation and reason were often inseparable from one another. Insanity became a figure of speech for all types of erratic, pagan, or unchristian, and, by the lights of the church, not fully rational behavior. Therefore, the lawgivers spoke of "pagan insanity," "Jewish madness," "Arian insanity," "barbaric irrationality." Faced with these threats of a disorder which seemed like cosmic madness, the church ruled that "natural law, starting with the origin of rational creatures, as it was said above, remains immovable."[64] St. Thomas seems to have said the final words on the relations between sanity and law. "As in man reason rules and commands the other powers, so all the natural inclinations belonging to the other powers must needs be directed according to reason. Wherefore it is universally right for all men that all their inclinations should be directed to reason." Finally, St. Thomas said, "it is . . . evident that natural law is nothing else than the rational creature's participation in the eternal law."[65] Irrational creatures fell short of full participation in natural law.

## COMMONS AND CUSTOMS: THE INSANE IN ENGLISH AND IRISH LAW

The concept of natural law and the specific laws of the canons were operant throughout Christendom. All canon lawyers in medieval Europe and England turned to Roman law whenever the "ius novum" contained no provision for a case. One nation alone is famous for resisting

Roman law during its formative period and this is the nation which provides so many of our own legal antecedents, England. The English protested that theirs were not the laws of Rome, yet, as many canonists have pointed out, they were heavily influenced, first, through the canon law operant throughout the English ecclesiastical system and, second, through the influence of the greatest medieval English jurists, Lanfranc, Vacarius, Glanville (who was the least influenced by Roman law), and Bracton. From the period of Vacarius in the twelfth century to that of Bracton, the formative period of English common law, the influence of Rome persisted.

Although much of English law for the insane is remarkably similar in tone and temper to Roman and canon law, there are some major differences. These lie in the mode of procedure and in the choice of the individual responsible for the affairs of the mad. Ultimately, the king, so omnipotent in England's laws, was the final guardian. The chief procedural difference between English and Roman law was that guilt was attached to the insane despite the fact that they were not held responsible for their acts. Since they were guilty without responsibility, they had to be tried and then pardoned by the king. This was the common practice, although lunatics could be subsequently restrained for the duration of their insanity in order to protect others.

In civil matters, English law was often even more stringent than Roman law. Any harm brought about by a madman or infant was liable to civil action for damages, because the consideration of intent was nonexistent during this period in English legal history. Damage was damage and the offender had to make reparation for his injurious actions. Instead of exculpating the madman, the English law extended mercy by occasionally lessening the punishment to which he was sentenced.

Yet, in the matters of property and maintenance, English law was particularly scrupulous with regard to the mad. English law, by the time of Henry III, divided the mad into two types: idiots and lunatics. Both were in the care of guardians, though the law, in force from the time of Edward III and possibly even Edward II, indicates that guardians of lunatics seem to have been entitled to some profit on the care of their charges' properties and so this duty was desirable. The guardians of lunatics were especially forbidden to take profit and their function was regarded as a duty. In both cases, however, waste of the profits was prohibited and return of property to the mad when sanity was restored was enjoined. In the case of lunatics and madmen the "king shall have the custody of the lands" but in the first he is allowed to "take profits without waste," "after their death, restoring them to their right heirs."[66] In the second case, "the king is to provide that the lunatic and his family are properly maintained out of the income of his estate, and the residue is to be handed over to him upon his restoration to sanity, or should he die without having recovered his wits, is to be administered by the ordinary for the good of his soul; but the king is to take nothing for his own use."[67] Apparently profit taking was not uncommon in the cases of idiots, and not until the time of Blackstone were idiots accorded protection by being granted the legal status of lunatics.

In almost every society we have mentioned, the insane were regarded exclusively as deficient, lacking in reason, sense, will, knowledge. This was not universally true. Especially the barbaric customal laws sometimes regarded the mad as weak or incompetent and yet simultaneously considered them gifted with a strange knowledge and strength. In these societies the laws for the mad treat their subjects as taboo; they fear but revere them. It may be that this pagan attitude underlies that balance of protection, privilege and deprivation which is the foundation of all major legal systems which deal with insanity. Certainly we can find no more stark or stripped view of insanity than the one which emerges in a code of customal law. Perhaps the most fascinating and voluminous body of Western customal law on the subject of insanity is the *Senchus Mor*, a late collection of early Irish customs.

From the laws of the *Senchus Mor*, we discover that early Irish society countenanced the possibility that madness could be supernatural and the mad are, therefore, respected, perhaps because they are close to nature, and are often accorded an elevated status. They are also divided according to the origin of their madness. There are: a geilt, a lunatic; a fulla, a lunatic who has had the magic wisp thrown at him; an abloire, a buffoon or a low fool, presumably an idiot. Irish customal law showed a degree of reverence for fools because, in some cases, the folly was seen as divinely initiated, for better or for worse. In most cases, however, the mad are discussed in terms startlingly like those of Roman law except that some of the similes are different. We hear echoes in the law that "no contracts are made binding on fugitives from a tribe who are proclaimed . . . adulteresses, idiots, dotards, fools, persons without sense, madmen."[68] The laws clearly enjoined guardianship: "In the case of fools, madmen, idiots, and dumb people, their persons were exempt from distress, but their guardians could be distrained . . ."[69] The tribe and family were supposed to maintain mad people, and the insane were unable to accept profits. For fostering them, however, their kinsfolk or guardians were rewarded. "In the case of the connection of mockery, of a lunatic, or a mad woman, neither of them is entitled to any share of profits or losses; the person who united them for fun and the sensible adult before whom it was done, are bound to foster the offspring, if offspring ensue of it, and bear their crimes and become their security. Their eric [body fine] and their legacy belong to the king and the church and the tribe."[70] We are also told that a madwoman's "rights precede all rights." These laws which originated in the judgments of the pagan Brehons, prior to or contemporary with the Christian era, were revived by St. Patrick and were generally recognized in Ireland until the reign of James I, in the seventeenth century.

Not only these laws but also the Roman and canon laws of insanity remained in use for a surprisingly long period, even into the modern era. Some of their force and much of their intent and emphasis survive today in the major legal considerations of juridical capacity, compulsion, inability to distinguish right from wrong, and unimputability. Throughout history the insane have, in the rules of law, shared that special form of privilege reserved for those who are treated with simultaneous condescension and solicitude. Yet these two apparently contradictory attitudes are actually two sides of one coin. Because of the legal protection granted to the insane, because of their immunity, they have been among the most feared segments of the populace. As men and women who have an acknowledged ability to act without responsibility for their actions, to harm without being legal agents of injury, the mad remained in a gray area of disputed jurisdiction. Ironically, the guardians and custodians were better understood and more suspiciously supervised than were the mad and ill-defined wards in their care.

# CHAPTER IV

## BAREFOOT AND BREADLESS
### *The Social Condition of the Insane*

> Barefoot and Breadless: beg they of
> no man.
>
> —LANGLAND, *Piers Plowman*

Since the advent of the "Gutenberg Galaxy," that nearly cosmic spinoff of the print explosion, we of the twentieth century can hardly conceive of lost history. With an almost religious faith, we are committed to a belief that not only is "the truth" discoverable but also that it is recoverable. If only we exhume the contents of enough newspaper morgues, scan enough bibliographies, thumb through all of the catalogues of the world's libraries, brush the dust from all the manuscripts lost and found, we must surely compile a full record of the past. Fresh with the glow of democratic light shed on the minutest routines of ordinary, and especially underprivileged, people, we remain convinced that the dead of past ages shared our fascinations and so left us a written account of all the social problems and human interests akin to our own.

Perhaps it is a testimony to the nobility of the human intellect that historical skepticism, scientific sophistication and even the well-worn cliché that the Middle Ages is a vast period of lost or nonexistent record cannot shake our faith that somewhere the truth lies fixed on a musty page. Nothing could be less true. The results are not in yet, of course, and, happily, there are still many manuscripts and documents which lie buried in the great metropolitan and provincial libraries of Europe. Yet we now know enough to have a sense of what is unknowable and why. Daily diaries of ordinary men and women are largely nonexistent because the average man and woman could not write and, even if they had been able, they had not the leisure to do so. Analytical inquiries into the plights of women, children, serfs, the poor, lepers and madmen are scarce in the extreme for several reasons. Among these illiteracy and lack of leisure again rank high, but disinterest in such subjects constitutes the principal explanation for the dearth of materials.

This disinterest was dictated by a hierarchy of values which insisted that the ordinary, the powerless and the irredeemable were simply less important than the heroic, the ruling classes and the salvageable.

Furthermore, attitudes toward these groups were, particularly in the popular mind, fixed and codified. Social behavior followed the dogma of the codes. Women were tempters and spiritually and intellectually unfit to rule, Eves, if they were not saints or martyrs. Children, unless they were miraculous or supernatural, were dear innocents but, fundamentally, mere offshoots of their lineal ancestors, whose roles they would one day assume. The poor and the serfs were poor and serviceable because, as some medieval philosophers were wont to say, "God made them so." Lepers and madmen, who fell into one social and moral group, were reflections of their diseases, which were either tests of martyrdom, purgations or punishments for sin.

It would be folly to say that these attitudes never changed or that there are no remaining records or documents. Since neither culture nor time is static, we do find exceptions to the law of unwritten record. Toward the end of the thirteenth century, social mobility increased, literacy became more widespread and austere religious sects proliferated. Then a growing interest in the lives of ordinary citizens and a sympathy for the disenfranchised were manifested in an increase of written records. But record keeping was dependent upon more than mere institutions and historical changes. It has always been the passion of individuals who were eccentric in their desire to chronicle and describe, or of rulers who valued the preservation of history. These figures, like genius itself, may appear in any century. The records mentioned here are, of course, the official documents which describe governmental or institutional treatment of the insane. Theoretical treatises in medicine, ecclesiastical doctrine, and law, all describing the insane and their diseases, were obviously plentiful, but records of the real and popular attitudes toward the insane are scarce. To expose the actual, rather than the theoretical and ideal, social treatment of the insane, we must reconstruct the concealed facts from those largely fragmented sources which are currently available. For this reason the concept of record must be more flexible and all-inclusive. Three major questions confront the modern inquirer into the general social attitudes toward the insane of the Middle Ages. Where can we find the records of the actual treatment of the insane? How are we to evaluate the accuracy of these records? What are the general attitudes they reveal?

The first question is answered partially by five well-known accounts of individual cases of insanity and the social response to it. Two of these—the English mystic Margery Kempe's account of her own "sicknesse" and the historian Froissart's chronicle of King Charles VI's illness —are more complete than the others. The other three are the poet Hoccleve's apparently autobiographical verse about his melancholy, the "autobiographical" drawings of an Italian priest, and the account of Hugo van der Goes's mental disease, written by his fellow monk Gaspar Offhuys.[1] Confirming the general absence, lateness and peculiar importance of accounts of insanity, all of these descriptions appear in the fourteenth and fifteenth centuries and all are devoted to important and unusual people—a famous mystic, a king of France, a self-conscious

poet, a notably literate monk. Only Margery is illiterate
and of quite modest economic origins, and her biography
was dictated to another, who "took it down." Skepticism
about either the objectivity or the popular nature of the
descriptions of social response found in these works is
clearly in order.

As a scientific or historical control against which we
may check popular attitudes and treatment, we have two
other types of sources besides the theoretical materials
discussed in the earlier chapters. These are fictional works
featuring mad heroes or heroines or merely reflecting upon
insanity itself, and non-fictional materials. The latter category is a grab bag of hospital records, town records,
charters and folk maxims. Each of these types also pre-
sents problems. The fictional material, often most revealing and even influential, is, nevertheless, bound to a series
of literary conventions and sometimes originates as a
mere imitation or variation of an earlier work on the same
characters or theme. The hospital and town records are
usually fragmentary, often propagandistic, in response to
influences of which we are not entirely aware, and frequently report events the circumstances of which have
been lost. The folk maxims suffer as historical sources
from the old cliché that they "lose in translation," translation not only of the language but of the folk and the
folkways. Despite the fact that we must grudgingly con-
struct a general view from this assemblage of historical
tatters, we find that a coherent image does emerge from
the accretion of records.

The most cogent discussions are the accounts of the
madness of representative figures. Happily, the mad in
these accounts are a cross section of medieval society and
they may be seen as a metaphor of the figures on the
famous diagram of the wheel of fortune, representing men
in the process of social and moral descent from the
empyrean position of king to the lowliest position of beggar. Three of the figures are also members of the re-

nowned "three orders" of medieval society. Hugo van der Goes belongs to the *oratores* (the prayers), Charles VI is one of the *bellatores* (the fighters) and Margery Kempe, despite her bourgeois station, is one of the *laboratores* (the workers). In anti-modern but true medieval fashion, let us begin with the king.

The French fourteenth-century historian Froissart wrote a long chronicle of the reign of King Charles VI of France, who, during his kingship, suffered three episodes of insanity. The first occurred when the king, against the advice of his physicians, set out on a military campaign. Even before his expedition, the king had been physically ill, feverish and exhausted from his labors. The court physicians pleaded with Charles to rest so that he could "gette himself . . . helthe or recovery of his last sicknesse," but Charles replied that he was well, in order to give courage to his men. The doctors' advice so disturbed the king that he could not recover. Finally, in the city of Le Mans, the king acceded to the advice of his physicians and counselors and rested for three weeks, during which time he was so "sore vexed with the fever" that his doctors warned his brother and uncles, "We ensure you ye do evil to travel the kyng, for he is in no good state to ryde."

Ride he did and the day he chose for his departure was "marvelous hot," the sun in his "chief force," so that Charles, weak with fever and overwork, was not "perfectly whole all that season." "He was feble in his brayne and heed and did eat or drink but lytell, and nygh dayly was in a hote fever . . . malencoly, and his spirytes sore troubled and travailed," but his physicians could not heal him.

By report, Froissart heard that, as the king rode along, "a great signification fell to him, by which, if he had done well, he should have called his counsel about him and well advised himself before he had gone further." This was the omen.

Sodaynly there came to the kynge a poore man, bare headed, bare legged and barefooted, and on his body a poore whyte cote; he semed rather to be a foole than wyse, and boldely sodaynly he toke the brydell of the kynges horse in his handes, and stopped the horse, and sayd: syr kyng, ryde no further forward for thou arte betrayed. These wordes entred into the kynges head, whereby he was worse dysposed in his helthe than he was before, so that his herte and his blode was moved. Than the Kynges servauntes [struck] and made no more of his wordes than of a fooles spekyng, which was foly as dyverses men sayde. For at the leste they shulde have better examyned the man, and to have seen if he had ben a naturall foole or no, and to have knowen fro when he came; but they dyde nat so, but lefte hym be-hynde, and he was never sene after to any mannes knowledge. . . .[2]

The shock and horror caused by the incident apparently left an impression upon the mind of the king, who re-garded it as an omen of evil. Even Froissart clearly indi-cates that God ordained this vision as part of a psychologi-cal scourge of pride, for he refers to Nebuchadnezzar, who, in his highest estate, was cast down from glory by the "ordainer of all things" who "aparelled this sayde king in such wyse that he lost his wit and reign and was seven year in that estate and lyved by acornes and maste" until the penance was complete. Only then did God restore Nebuchadnezzar's wit and memory. Froissart tells us that the sickness which followed hard upon the king's encounter with the poor man was a fitting consequence of the king's pride, for he ought not to have ridden out against the advice of his physicians, in his weakened state, on such a glaringly hot day.

What followed was an incident of paranoia, or, as medieval men would have called it, a "triumph of the

imagination over reason." One of the pages in the king's
retinue dropped his spear on that of another with a great
clash and the king, instantly recalling the image of the
poor man and the dire words about betrayal, began to
believe that he was pursued by his enemies, who wished
to slay him, and "with that abusyon, he fell out of his
wytte by febleness of his heed . . . having no knowledge
of any man; believing that he was in battle enclosed with
his enemies" and laying about him with his sword, "he
cared not where, and cryed and sayd: On, on upon these
traitours." The king, Froissart tells us, was in such a
"frenzy" that he did not know his own relatives who cried
out, "the kynge is nat in his right mind."

The men at arms surrounded the violent king and saved
both themselves and his honor by falling before each
stroke of his sword until he wearied himself and was, at
last, restrained by one of his favorite knights, who held
him while he was stripped of his weapons. They then
removed his jacket to refresh him and returned him to
Le Mans by horse litter. The reactions of his kinsmen were
confused. They were "sore abayssed, and wyste nat what
to say or do." Yet this frenetic was a king and so their
humiliation was alloyed with pity and a liberal dose of
philosophy, that "the French kyng, who as at that tyme
was reputed for the moste noble and puyssant kynge in
all Crystendome, fell so sodaynly out of his minde without remedy, but as God wolde." The lesson is biblical and
a doctrinal commonplace: "Lo, how the mighty have
fallen"; "Beware the sin of pride."

Also because he was a king, Charles received the best
medical attention. The physicians who "have much ado
with hym" pointed out that "the kyng of long tyme had
engendred the same malady." They had expected, after
all, and even predicted an incident of this sort, "for we
knew well that the wekenes of his brayne wold sore trouble hym, and at last shewe itself." When the royal household gathered by his bedside the next morning, the king

was unable to recognize any of its members "and loked straungely on them, and had lost clene the knowledge of them." His doctors prescribed a careful diet to ameliorate his frenetic condition, and rest. His relatives offered constant prayers for his recovery and recover he did. But it was noted that he was a type, weakened in the brain by overexposure to heat and exhaustion, naturally given, in any case, to an immoderate temperament alternating between frenzy and melancholy. Predictably, he suffered several other attacks of mild disturbance and, finally, in 1394, the king was again afflicted with insanity.

This time overindulgence in the pleasures and pastimes at the festivities of Abbeville upset his psychic balance and "he fell agayne into his maladye of frenzy, in like manner as he had been the yere before." The king's sickness was concealed from the populace as fully as possible and he was conveyed by night to a secluded castle.

This second illness had some serious political consequences, for the French people began to suspect that the character of their king was an unstable one. They perceived the pattern which the physicians, with their greater sophistication and acuity, had detected so much earlier. Excess was the cause, everyone said. Charles was immoderate in his actions and habits and his inherent weakness of the brain was, thus, easily exploited and developed into a full-fledged insanity. The physicians tried their remedies again, but even they were skeptical about the effect or permanence of their efforts; the king's problem was a chronic one. The second cure, Froissart indicated, was effected principally by the noble deeds of Charles's queen, who gave "much almesses, and . . . many pilgrimmages for the kynge, and caused general processions to be made in Paris." Medical, physical and spiritual remedies were all tried, but the spiritual were the most successful. The noteworthy elements in this episode are the acceptance of the chronic nature of the king's disease and, even more outstanding, the great comfort and care devoted to him even in the worst rages of his illness. Of course, he merited this therapy and concern because he was the king, a hereditary ruler and a wealthy man who did not have to endure the outrages and deprivations of the poverty-stricken mad.

Froissart's analysis of the causes of the king's illnesses is repetitive, consistent and all-inclusive. The frenzy to which the king was chronic prey was "manifestly the work of God, whose punishments are severe, to make his creatures tremble."[3] His madness was a "period of penitence" and also the result of the "great influence from Heaven . . . and, as some say, from his own fault." The influence from heaven was both moral and physical, for the hot sun, shining upon a "constitution" physically ill suited to heat, promoted a fever of the brain as well as the body, a medical fact of the day which serves as a metaphor for the whole condition of the nation, when Froissart notes that, "being the chief, every part of the government suffered; for, in like manner when the head of a man is sick, his other members are not painless."

The physicians were berated for their neglect of a physical constitution leading to frenzy, and they declared that his first illness proceeded from emotional and physical causes: "the alarm in the forest, and by inheriting too much of his mother's weak nerves."

The bias of the priests and of the king's enemies was moral; the king was a supporter of the antipope, a physical overindulger, and the rest and diet prescribed by the physicians could be of little service because "there could not be any remedy applied, nor any amendment expected, since God willed it should be so." Gossip of the schemers and the general populace, however, ran to plot and treachery during the king's first illness. "The event was spoken of very differently: some said that the king, to ruin the kingdom of France, had been poisoned, or bewitched, the morning before he left Mans." The plot theory was, however, finally discredited by investigation.

Three episodes of frenzy were explored at length by Froissart, and each occurred under slightly different circumstances, but overexhaustion, overindulgence, hot weather and genetic disposition were factors common to all. The onset of the illness occurred under new circumstances each time, but the symptoms were the same. In each case, his "senses were quite gone," he "showed no symptoms of acquaintance or affection, but rolled his eyes round in his head without speaking to anyone." He was harrowed by fever, heat, hallucinations, insomnia and amnesia, anorexia.

The social response to the king in his illness stands in marked contrast to that accorded the madman who accosted the king in the first episode which provoked his insanity. "As the man finished his speech, the men at arms beat him soundly on his hands," and then "suffered him to run off, without paying any attention to what he had said, thinking he was some madman, for which they were by many afterwards greatly blamed and disgraced: they ought at least to have arrested him, to have examined if he were really mad, and to learn why he had uttered such words, and whence he had come." The homespun clothing, the bare head, the naked feet of the prophet of doom were, for the king's men, sure signs of madness. The forest setting, the poor clothing and unmannerly behavior were socially and, therefore, spiritually disorderly. Violent treatment of the madman was condemned not because he was pitiable—indeed, it seemed appropriate to treat a mad creature so—but because it neglected sensible interrogation before the beating. If the man were mad, his information would be inaccurate, but if he were sane, he would have valuable political news. The kings' men-at-arms' treatment was just for a mere madman but careless behavior if the man could have offered useful information.

The king was indeed more violent than the forest madman, but he was carried to the castle of Creil, "which has good air, and is in a rich country on the river Oise."

There he was treated by the great physician Master William de Harsley, who administered medicines and rest, to no avail because God, "to correct him, punished him with this rod of frenzy." Eventually medicine and prayer restored the king's "intellects," but the most effective cure was one reminiscent of Arnold of Villanova's seals. A wax figure "in the shape of the king" was sent with a taper to the "church at Haspres in Hainault [where lies] the canonized body of Saint Aquaire in a rich shrine of silver. This saint is celebrated for the cures he has performed on those afflicted with madness, and on that account is much visited from all parts." "A similar offering was made to Saint Hermier in Rouais, who has the reputation for curing madness, and wherever there were saints that were supposed to have efficacy, by their prayers to God, in such disorders, thither were sent offerings from the king, with much ceremony and devotion." The king's second frenzy, brought on by heat and overindulgence, was most effectively treated by religious acts of charity and small doses of rest, and his third rage, by now expected in moments of stress, was the result of emotional distraction over political events.

As an intelligent historian, devoted to the exploration of all phenomena, Froissart proposed and analyzed all of the remarks about the king's madness. He noted that various interest groups assigned different causes and significations to the king's illness and that each tried its cure for its own diagnoses, yet Froissart himself arrived at his own amalgam of causes and meanings. The king had a poor heredity, a nervous and overheated constitution. His spiritual disposition led him to disregard his God-given nature and to overindulge his appetites and his worldly desires and he was punished for so doing. The result was a psychosomatic illness—overheating of the body and brain, fever and mania which were treated in their secondary or physical manifestations by medical therapy, and in their primary or psycho-spiritual manifestations by prayer and offerings of sympathetic magical character.

From this account it is apparent that kings and beggars might both suffer madness, but that society treated one with care, the second with abuse, and that a monarch's state of intellect was inseparable from the divine plan of history. However much pity was expended upon the illness of Charles, and there was great sympathy from his friends, that sympathy could not prevent distrust. The Duke of Lancaster especially testified his sorrow, and said to the knights near his person: "On my faith, it is great pity, for he showed himself a man of courage, with strong inclinations to do good." He must add, "There is an end to this, for he will never again have that confidence he before enjoyed put in him." "That is true enough," said those who heard him, "and the kingdom of France seems likely to fall into much trouble."

Margery of Kempe of Lynn, daughter of John Brunham, mayor of Lynn, was married to John Kempe in 1393. While Charles VI of France was suffering from his frenzy and riding to battle, Margery was pursuing the path to a mystical union which was to lead her into a frenzy very different in its appearance from the mysterious illness of which Charles was to be so often cured. She too suffered insanity, but her "madness," as she so willingly called it, was a fortunate martyrdom which she endured without ambivalence and understood without ambiguity. One of a long line of mystics who prayed that they might be visited with a purgation of pain, Margery welcomed her noisy "fits" as purifications from sin and irrational possessions by the force of divine love. An early liberated woman, Margery bound her husband to a vow of chastity and celibacy, left her fireside and wandered over England, Germany, Spain, Italy and Jerusalem, to the sites of the mystical saints and the pilgrimage shrines. She orchestrated her voyages with weepings, wailings and shrieking and, toward the end of her life, God bade her seek a literate person to write down her experiences as she "told" them so that the book might serve the purpose of holy instruction.

Margery dated her conversion to mystical devotion from the day on which she understood that "our Lord with great bodily sickness [had touched her with his hand] where through she lost reason and her wits a long time till our Lord by grace restored her a-geyn . . ." Later, when she received "inspiration of the Holy Ghost," she wept and sobbed and "could not herself tell the grace that she felt, it was so heavenly, so high above her reason and her bodily wits," so high indeed that mere men often doubted her sanity.

Margery's sickness was a visitation of pain which lasted eight weeks. It afflicted various portions of her anatomy including her head and her back and she "feared that she would lose her wit through it." This illness, which Margery called "God's punishment for her sins," left her subject to great fits of weeping and shrieking, especially during mass. Her crying and moaning increased to such a degree that "priests dare not give her the eucharist openly in church but in the priory chapel at Lynn away from the hearing of the people."[4] "And in that chapel she had so high contemplation and so much dalliance of our lord, in as much as she was put out of church for his love, that she cried when she was given the eucharist, as if her body would be parted asunder, so that two men held her arms till her crying was ceased, for she could not bear the abundance of love that she felt in the precious sacrament which she steadfastly believed was very God and Man in the form of bread." One monk refused to come into the chapel when she was there, so that she had to make confession and take the eucharist in the church. Since she had a letter from the Lord of Canterbury announcing that her visions were holy and commanding that she be given the sacrament when she required it, the priest had to give her the sacrament. Her noisy seizures proved an infuriating distraction to the other parishioners, for, during the

mass, she "sobbed, roared, and cried, and spreading her
arms abroad, said with a loud voice, 'I die, I die,' that
many men there wondered and marveled what ailed
her."[5]

Margery continued to carry on in this manner for ten
years, and during this time she remained convinced that
her seizures were a special blessing from God. Finally,
even Margery began to weary of waiting for the fulfillment of her religious longings. Unfortunately, not all of
the people who heard Margery's performances shared her
enthusiasm for her manifestations of love and their skepticism contributed to her restlessness when she said:

> I begin to madden, for love governeth me and not
> reason. I run with hasty course wherever thou wilt.
> I bow, Lord, that they who see me are annoyed and
> distressed, not knowing me drunken with thy love.
> Lord, they cry, "Lo, yon mad man crieth in the
> streets."[6]

Margery's contrast between reason and love is central
to her belief that there is a divine madness, a madness
which is insane on earth and divinely sane in heaven. Yet
she recognizes her original illness as a scourge, divinely
instigated, nevertheless, a disease of purgation. Her neighbors and the local clergymen have the more predictable
and immediate response. One friar maintains that "sche
hath a devyl whythinne her." The townspeople who are
friendly toward her are less theoretical and highly practical, for they form a delegation to tell her, in understated
terms, that "it were more easy to her to go out of the
town than to abide therein, so many people are against
her."

Ignoring the mystical interpretation of her seizures and
regarding her, not as modern mystics, but as modern ra-
tionalists, who share the fears and instinctive responses of
medieval men, we are likely to see her as a maniac, a

paranoid schizophrenic, seized alternately by weeping, sobbing and delusions of persecution. Although she, as the wife of an alderman and the daughter of a mayor, is accorded certain economic and social privileges, she is not of royal blood and some of her delusions are, in fact, clear-eyed assessments of social attitudes. Her behavior is disruptive, and eccentric, infuriating and terrifying. Her belief in her own powers and her special grace did triumph, however, at least with the church. Even some townsfolk believed in her gifts and one of her little miracles was the soothing of a madwoman, an act which suggested that she had that sympathy with insanity which was the attribute of the saints of the mad. The church's treatment of Margery stands in stark contrast to the townsfolk's behavior toward the other madwoman, a more commonplace citizen.

In church Margery met a man who was wringing his hands in sorrow, and when she inquired about the source of his misery, he told her that his "wife was newly delivered of a child and she was out of her minde. 'And, dame,' he seyeth, 'she knoweth not me nor none of her neighbors. She roareth and crieth so that she maketh folk evil afeared. She will both smite and bite and therefore is she manacled on her wrists.'"[7] With his consent, Margery visited the woman and saw that she was "aliened of her wit." When the townsfolk approached the woman, she "wold not suffryn them to touch her. . . . She cried and gaped as if she would eat them and said she saw many devils about them." About Margery she saw angels and she was comforted by Margery's presence, but she reverted to her hysterical behavior, what we would call postpartum hysteria, as soon as Margery left her side. Her roaring and crying both night and day antagonized and frightened the people and most would "not suffer her to dwell among them." Thus, they removed her to "the fartherst end of the town into a chamber so that the people should not hear her crying. And there was she bound hands and feet

with chains of iron that she should smite nobody."
Margery prayed every day to God that he should, "if it
were his will, restore her wits again." God answered, "She
shall fare right well," and so she did. After purification
in church, the woman was cured and restored to the rights
of the community. We are told that God gave the illness
and God took it away, but man must intercede with God
and, finally, cleanse the possessed of the pollution of
madness.

The manacles were used only to protect the woman
from herself as well as to protect others from her, but her
incarceration and subsequent neglect by her neighbors are
marks of the unalloyed terror and hostility the insanity of
a commoner could evoke from fellow citizens. In Margery's
behavior we see the bias of the religious; in the townspeople's, we see the popular and unexamined response.
We may ask ourselves why she was not committed to an
asylum and our answer will, of course, be that there were
no local asylums during this period. We may ask why no
physician was summoned and we shall realize that medical care was rare and not for the ordinary soul in the
hinterlands in the fourteenth century. In English rural
areas in the fourteenth century, mental-health care was
everybody's business when the family of the victim did
not provide it. If the madwoman seems to have been
abused in a peculiarly medieval way, we must ask ourselves how we treat the criminally insane. In this story,
the prayers of a woman graced redeemed the soul of a
woman cursed. Margery's calm presence is therapeutic but
the real cure is effected by the heavenly physician, as
medieval authors liked to call God.

The three remaining figures of whose madness we have
lengthy accounts are all artists and their insanity belongs
to the artistic tradition. Whether or not they experienced
temporary manias, they were all, temperamentally, children of Saturn, or melancholics. Perhaps because they
were melancholics primarily, rather than maniacs, their

madness is less dramatic, more problematical. Opicinus de Canistris, who flourished between 1296 and about 1350, was born in Pavia, a contemporary of Dante, Giotto and Petrarch. His history survives largely because of his work, a volume of remarkably large drawings, two tracts and a great deal of written commentary, part of which is an account of his "illness." The details of his life history are to be found mainly in the writing on a "series of enormous sheets and drawings."[8]

From the age of ten, his future as a cleric in the church was determined. His major talent and pleasure lay in drawing, but he also attended classes in medicine. He worked as a teacher in Genoa and then, to increase his income, he learned the art of manuscript illustration. His studies were interrupted by his father's death, but he received sufficient support to complete his religious studies and achieve ordination. Partially due to the excommunicated state of Pavia, he came under constant political attack and later, for other reasons, pressure from his creditors. For "unknown reasons" he was investigated and tried, an ordeal which tired him and produced great strain.

During this period, he became ill and recorded a dream. "I was in Venice, a town I had known only from descriptions. When I opened my eyes I felt as if I had awoken from eternal sleep and was born again. I had forgotten everything and could not recall how the world outside looked." He also had a vision of a vase—"canistra" in Latin —in the clouds and noted that he was mute, "paralyzed in [my] right hand and had lost, in a miraculous way, a large part of my memory of letters (or learnings)."

Despite the fact that his right hand was paralyzed, Opicinus, who now could not write the chancery documents, a job he disliked, was able to execute with this same right hand twenty-seven enormous drawings, which were miraculously dictated to him and were produced "without human assistance." The pattern of dissociation recorded by Opicinus, the irrational combinations in the twenty-seven drawings and the cleric's description of his own illness and subsequent life led the art historian–psychiatrist Ernst Kris to diagnose the "illness" as schizophrenia combined with an obsessive psychosis and hysteria. The drawings themselves are of particular interest. One of the map of Italy is almost engulfed by the body of the Virgin and this body shows a remarkable and almost blasphemous interest in female anatomy and fetal positions. Texts on the drawings show that the author's partial purpose was to prove his own legitimacy, and these texts were juxtaposed with the feet of the Virgin, which are labeled "husband" and "wife." With depictions and legends of eternal damnation, the limner mentions high ecclesiastic honors for himself and, at the same time, the notion that these honors portend evil. In these works there is frequent evidence of that "horror vacui" so typical of the drawings of both ancient and modern schizophrenics, and many patterns which are completely untypical of any other medieval art known.[9] Tiny figures, for example, appear inside other figures, and without the standard theological justifications of sheltering or divine birth. The author is, in his pictorial autobiography, obsessed with creating a personal system of the universe which bears no relation to standard theology or cosmogony and is written over, drawn over, then overwritten again, producing an image of overcrowding, obsession, a terrible disorderly order comparing and, at once, contrasting the benefits of power and the damnation of advancement. The language and the associations in what proclaims itself a religious and/or cosmic work are idiosyncratically personal and interior, so that they bear no relation to either doctrinal schemata or generally comprehensible visions of the universe.

Opicinus never mentioned insanity in his account. He was convinced, perhaps even more than Margery, that his illness was a divine purgation. What is more interesting is that there is no account of any monastic ostracism. No doubt his obsession with divine possession and the subsequent devotion to a holy mission helped to assure his continuing acceptance in a community of the religious. His sickness was passive rather than violent and, indeed, a lesser degree of melancholy was commonly considered the special destiny of intellectuals and clerks, so that he did not exercise the disruptive influence of either Margery or King Charles VI.

Almost two centuries later, in 1475, the then well-known painter Hugo van der Goes entered a monastery as a lay brother. There he partook of certain privileges, notably eating and drinking with noble visitors, which aroused the jealousy of another brother, Gaspar Offhuys, who later took a savage pleasure in describing in detail his "curious mental illness."[10] Apparently the artist was, even before his illness, given to fits of melancholy, but his gloomy thoughts, which arose from his despair of achieving his artistic aims, never overwhelmed him until he took a certain journey. Then he began to say "incessantly that he was damned and judged eternally to be damned and, unless restrained forcefully by a bystander, would harm himself physically and lethally." In Brussels, the abbot saw the analogy between Hugo's illness and King Saul's and so prescribed music and pleasant spectacles, but Hugo did not recover for a long time.

Gaspar, less charitable and more self-interested than the abbot, discussed the causes of Hugo's illness and concluded that it was either natural in origin, arising from melancholic meats, the drinking of strong wines, from passions of the spirit, namely care, sadness or excessive study or fear, or imposed by God, who wished to save the artist from the sin of pride by means of a "humbling illness." Neither diagnosis led to Hugo's expulsion. He had a ready-made hospital and the job of the religious was either to assist in the cure of his illness and thus purge him of worldly disease, or to preserve him while God chastised

him so that he might survive as a living example of the
spells of pride and the joys of humility. Unfortunately, he
did not survive for very long and he remained temperamentally melancholic. He was judged as a sinner but
charitably judged. To those who cared for him, virtue was
the prize of charity. Their martyrdom, to read Gaspar,
was their farsighted tolerance of pride and overindulgence.

The toils of Saturn, melancholic fits, were the lot of
another contemporary of Hugo, the English poet Thomas
Hoccleve. Hoccleve, in his poetic letter to a friend, described himself as sick and crackbrained, but denied his
friend's assertion that too much study had maddened him.
According to Hoccleve's complaint, his friends did desert
him during the period of his illness, for they found him
distasteful, uncommunicative, sometimes frightening, and
they chastised him for permitting or even causing attacks
of mental illness. Alternately convinced that madness was
his sad destiny, conferred by God, and that it was his
given temperament, Hoccleve fought against the standard
view that rigorous exercise of the intellect inevitably provoked insanity. Knowledge or pride in intellectual pursuits
as a cause of madness was a persistent theme from the
time of the Bible. In Acts, when Peter accused Paul of
being mad, he added, "Too much study hath made thee
mad."

In his *Male Regle*, Hoccleve described a sinful or excessive regimen, as the title of the poem suggests. He has
been obsessed with the flesh and the world, he tells the
reader, absorbed with the spending and getting of worldly
goods. He describes the symptoms of melancholy which,
according to his *Complaint*, began five years earlier in a
frenzy, characterized by "continual waking, moving and
casting about of eyes, raging, stretching and casting of
hands, moving and wagging of the head . . ." We cannot be certain that Hoccleve was really mad any more
than we can be certain that Chaucer, at the moment of
his introduction to the *Book of the Duchess*, is a genuine

melancholic. Both may be taking advantage of the convenient literary convention of the maddened lover or sinner. Nevertheless, their descriptions of the diseases from which they suffered are perfect replications of medical symptomatology. The causes of the illness were, for Hoccleve, moral. He has been punished by God for his sins, purged by a madness which begins in frenzy and ends in melancholy, a melancholy caused and cured by God, assisted by the poet's acts of penance. Hoccleve's forbidden knowledge is one of the major themes of Genesis. The rending of the veil has always been taboo and priests have maintained a monopoly over the divine mysteries, to some of which even they were denied access. This horror of probing the mysteries is apparent in ancient cultures and even lurks behind the encyclopedic pursuits of high medieval learning. The reinforcement of holy ignorance seems to re-emerge in full flower in the fourteenth century, which praises its sanctity. Although the divine fool does appear throughout the Middle Ages, he becomes an increasingly common figure who achieves his greatest stature in the Renaissance praises of folly.

In the Middle Ages there is a war between unholy ignorance and holy innocence. From the eleventh through the thirteenth century, the writers and scholars generally opted for learning. By the fourteenth century Chaucer presaged more serious praises of folly and recognized the religious taboos current among common folk when his stupid carpenter in the *Canterbury Tales* mouths, "O, blessed be the foolish man." By the fifteenth century the growing humanism seemed to place too great a burden on man to know and control his universe, and men retreated before the weight of freedom. It is in this period that a new emphasis on the virtues of the weak intellect reached its height. But the earlier protesting religious movements of the late fourteenth century also helped to lay the groundwork.

William Langland's *Piers Plowman* is a poem dedicated

to the poor, the ordinary, the simple of this world. The folk so heartily praised in his work include lunatics and lollers, who merit particular care and love. That they seldom received this care is also obvious from Langland's description of the places and conditions in which they were to be found:

And they want their wits, men and women both,
The which are lunatic lollers and lepers about,
And mad as the moon sits, more or less.
They care for no cold, nor counteth of heat.
and are moving after the moon, moneyless they walk,
with a good will, witless, many wide countries
Just as Peter did and Paul, save that they preach not,
nor make miracles, and many times it befalls that they
prophesy of the people, playing as it were
and to our sight, as it seems, since God hath the might
To give each man wit, wealth, and his health
and yet allows such to go so, it seems to my conscience
they are his apostles, such people, or as his secret
    disciples.
For he sent them forth moneyless, in a somer garment,
without bread and bag, as the book telleth . . .

.      .      .      .      .      .      .      .      .      .      .

Such manner of men, Matthew teaches us,
We should have them to house and help them when they
    come

.      .      .      .      .      .      .      .      .      .      .

Give them rich gifts and gold, for great lordes sake.

.      .      .      .      .      .      .      .      .      .      .

For under God's secret seal, their sins are hidden.[11]

Langland's madmen are poverty-stricken lunatics, whose sanity changes with the moon. They are gifted with the insight of the God-struck, whose minds, fixed on the impractical, impervious to life, often seem divinely inspired with visions of another world. God, who could have done otherwise, has chosen these men as his apostles, nomads or prophets, whose innocent infirmities offer the ordinary man the opportunity to win grace through charitable deeds. Their virtue abounds because they are God's chosen, whose sins are observed and even erased by divinely granted innocence, an innocence which is at the core of our belief that they are mad. These tribes or individuals, Langland tells us, wandered starving over the countryside, cutting innocent capers, conveying their visions. They were neglected, like other objects for charity, and Langland's passage is a plea for better, kinder treatment and maintenance of the insane, who so often found either food nor shelter, but lived with jeers and the hardship of overexposure to the raw English elements.

These tribes of wandering madmen were not peculiar to England. The convention of the ship freighted with madmen and cast adrift found a hospitable literary setting in the various fifteenth- and sixteenth-century books called "ships of fools."[12] The commonest treatment accorded to the ordinary madman of the twelfth through the fourteenth centuries was social ostracism. He was either set afloat on a ship of madmen, enclosed in a prison-like chamber located within a town wall, like the tower of fools in Caen or the *Narrenturm* (fools' tower) at Nuremberg, or simply driven away. The evidence for forceful banishment appears in a number of town records which, like the fourteenth-century French payrolls, cite money to be given to one "king of the ribaud's [ribalds]" for "beating Agnes the fool" or an order to requite one man for "driving out a fool counterfeiting a maniac."[13]

Not in the medical mind, but in the popular mind, insanity and idiocy were synonymous and there is a well-known but unsubstantiated maxim that the fool may have the fool's privilege of speaking freely since he is not held responsible for anything he says. Granted protection as an innocent plaything of nature and the king, the fool was often treated as the truth teller of the court. Though he might be beaten at the sovereign's will to "beat some sense into him," he was nevertheless feared and respected and expected to display certain talents. He was to be able to imitate or "ape" the voices and actions of others, as in the thirteenth-century *Tristant,* the author, Eilhart von Oberge, calls the fool, Tristant in disguise, a "rechte affe," a real ape. He is supposed to be able to leap high into the air, a natural gift of the maniac, as we find in the medical texts of the period.

With the fool, another figure, the wild man, shared a pagan genealogy and the apelike qualities of the subhuman mentality. Both the fool and the wild man were folk figures, both touched with a supernatural quality ascribed to pre-Christian, almost demonic origins, often lost to the members of the common village or the uncommon court. Their behavior was savage or "sauvage," and the medieval world, especially in Germany, had not lost its contact with earlier religions. The forest remained, for medieval Christians, the terrifying haunt of paganism, waiting to spring to life again. The old religions survived in the form of superstitions recorded by, among others, Caesarius of Heisterbach in the twelfth century and Geiler von Kaiserberg in the fifteenth century. The first described a wild horde who rode on stormy nights and on holidays of the dead. Led by the demon Herlikin (a former Germanic storm god, later to be demoted to the common harlequin), they ravaged the country, leaving a path strewn with irrational and violent deeds, symptomatic, for the populace, of demonic madness.[14] Insanity, then, came to be associated with the countryside, the wilderness, the natural state which had predated both Christianity or rational society and the city or civilized, culture. In ancient Greece the Bacchic cults and their Dionysiac madness were celebrated in the countryside and the strange association of disorder and irrationality with wilderness persisted throughout the Middle Ages. A thirteenth-century English lyric calls love a "strange madness that leads the idle man through the wilderness."

Yvain, the hero of a famous twelfth-century romance by Chrétien de Troyes, suffered a madness which later became the model for German, Italian, French and English romance descriptions of insanity through the fourteenth century. When he realized that he had broken a vow to his wife, Yvain felt a growing dissociation. He said that his heart and head were severed and felt that guilt would drive him mad. Finally, when he is publicly shamed and renounced by a messenger from his lady, his symptoms of alienation become flagrant. Yvain feels "a storm rise in his head," jumps up, races away from the court and town, stripping away the symbols of his nobility and his knighthood as he leaves behind his horse, his sword and, finally, his clothes. He lives in the forest like a wild man, killing animals with his bare hands, eating the meat raw, running from people. A forest-dwelling hermit sees him and recognizes him as a madman, for he has a noble face but a disordered appearance and he is naked. Abandonment of the court and uncivilized immodest behavior are understood by a courtly audience, the target of this literary work, as symbols and synonyms of insanity. Wildness within is wildness without. The disordered mind finds its proper habitat in the chaos beyond the walls of the court. Yvain was found, recognized as a nobleman and cured by solicitous ladies. Like the king of France, mad Charles VI, he had an exalted rank and a noble lineage and, therefore, the best private care. His return to sanity was seen as a return to civilized and even courtly behavior.

From Langland's and Chrétien's descriptions, which are merely samples covering a wide span of time and nation and language, but are, nevertheless, fairly representative samples, we may gather that the rural madman was a neglected and an often maltreated nomad, a starving and sometimes abused beggar. In the case of the nobleman, household care was forthcoming and the family served as guardians, calling in, when they could, both medical and religious aid. In the towns, the mad were in a somewhat different situation. Sometimes there were places of incarceration where madmen, particularly if they could not be claimed by a family, were confined. Large cities had standard places of confinement, sometimes mere towers where the mad raged in chains, sometimes hospitals—usually, until the fourteenth and fifteenth centuries, leprosaria and almshouses where the poor, the mad, the chronically ill, lived together. There is no substantial record of any attempt to do more than feed and shelter the insane in these hospitals. The medical treatments in the medical school treatises were administered to nobles or else to individual clerics. Monasteries, which sometimes acted as hostels for the mad, the sick and the poor, provided kinder treatment and sometimes administered some care, but, again, the real records are slim and we can judge only on the basis of the descriptions of a late Gaspar Offhuys or Margery Kempe. The practical attitude in large settlements and their institutions was the religious one, God will provide. Time and God alone could be the healers. For this reason, the hospital was merely a waiting room.

Although we hear of hospitals for the insane as early as the eighth and ninth centuries in the Arab countries, we hear of no European hospital in which the insane were segregated for care until the late fourteenth or early fifteenth century.[15] Some of the most complete of all the very sparse accounts of hospitals for the insane come from England. Mary Rotha Clay, in her study of medieval hospitals of England, noted: "Formerly all needy people were admitted into the hospital, mental invalids being herded together with those weak or diseased in body. From the chronicle of St. Bartholomews, Smithfield, we learn that in the twelfth century mad people were constantly received as well as the deaf, dumb, blind, palsied, and crippled."[16] St. Mary of Bethlehem (Bedlam) was the most famous refuge for the insane and a census of the hospital taken in 1403 showed a populace of six men "deprived of reason, *mente capti* [their minds seized], and three other sick, one a paralytic who had been lying in the hospital for over two years." Apparently the condition was general, for insane, notably those suffering from attacks of mania, are confined in many "general infirmaries." Holy Trinity at Salisbury received not only sick people but also women in childbirth and mad people ("furiosi"), who were to be kept, according to instructions "until their senses returned." A petition for the reformation of hospitals in 1414 noted that they were established partly "to maintain those who had lost their wits and memory (*hor de leurs sennes et mémoire*)."[17]

The question of making special provisions for the mad did not become a serious issue until 1369, when a person named Denton tried to found a hospital for "poor priests and others, men and women, who in that city suddenly fell into a frenzy and lost their memory." Apparently his cause was lost and later, in 1419, a bequest was made to the sick and insane of St. Mary de Bedlam. In 1437, a Patent Roll entry spoke of the "succour of demented lunatics and others" but revealed that cutbacks would be expected unless financial aid was made rapidly available.[18] Thus it was not until the late fifteenth century that these hospitals became more specialized and until the late seventeenth century that Bedlam had its present meaning, as a hospital for the insane. The continental situation was, in this instance, not in advance of the English. Madmen, the chronically ill, sometimes the expectant, were housed together with the merely poor.

What functions these hospitals for the insane finally served is not entirely clear, for we are told of "a churche of oure Ladye that is named Bedlam. And in that place are found many men that been fallyn oute of hir witt. And full honestly they been kept in that place: And sum been restored unto their wits and health again and sum been abiding there forever, for they have fallen so much out of themselves that it is uncurable unto Man."[19] Apparently the problems of the medieval hospitals for the insane were identical to our own. Cure was, at best, uncertain and the efficacy of hospitalization as a therapeutic, rather than a socially cosmetic, force, questionable.

When, in the late fifteenth and sixteenth centuries, hospitals for the exclusive care of the mad became more common phenomena, we of the twentieth century think we see a greater concern and a growing social conscience. We must, however, examine the purposes of these hospitals and the social concepts they represent before we can be convinced that our assumption is correct. Since larger groups participated in planning for the insane, there is more general concern. Instead of considering the problems of mental-health care a private issue, society now considered them a corporate responsibility. The government began to assume duties which the church or the family or the court had formerly overseen. Furthermore, instead of considering madness one of many physical and spiritual ills which were undifferentiable, these bodies of government came increasingly to consider madness a "special" disease, a disease which, Michel Foucault said, replaced leprosy as the major social stigma and obsession.[20]

Whether the increasing number of special institutions for the mad shows a greater humanity is problematic. Ironically, in one sense, the period of so-called "humanism" is a period of dwindling humaneness in its treatment of the mad because the hospitals were institutionalized isolation chambers—more custodial than therapeutic. The word "asylum," which does not come into currency as a word particularly connoting a madhouse until the eighteenth century, originally meant a place of refuge or a sanctuary. Presumably, the most humane function of the mental hospital was that it "secured" the madman and prevented him from being liable to the taxation, punishment, imprisonment or attack which might be the lot of a normal man. Yet hospitals classed most of the mad in one amorphous lump. They were not schizophrenics or manic-depressives; they were just "furiosi" or "amenti," lunatics or idiots, but really merely mad. As patients in governmental institutions, these mad people became wards of the state with all that implied. To be a ward of the state meant to be cared for, but also to be shamed, to be deprived of individuality and recognizable identity. In this sense, then, hospitalization for the mad meant institutionalized deprivation of self and self-determination.

Furthermore, for the general citizenry, these madhouses became tainted places to be feared, shunned, even despised. Later they came to be regarded as zoos and circuses, providing spectacles, hilarity and curiosities for onlookers. We know, for example, that, in later years, Blake, Hogarth, Pepys and others found "interesting" subjects in the madhouses which they portrayed with greater sympathy for the human condition than did the observers of 1815 who issued a House of Commons report that "the hospital of Bethlehem exhibit[s] lunatics for a penny every Sunday."[21]

The medieval church may have been kinder to the madman than was the seventeenth-century hospital. One nineteenth-century French archivist claimed that a number of twelfth-century churches had special structures resembling choir screens, which he believes were designed to contain the mad during the mass. There, he maintained, the mad were confined in a space where they could neither harm nor be harmed by the worshippers of the parish, and could, yet, be exposed to the spiritual benefits of the mass. I have not yet been able to confirm his assertion that structures were designed or used for this purpose, but an unexplained passage in Chrétien's *Yvain* puts into Guinevere's mouth the words that an unmannerly knight of her court has a temper and tongue so irredeemably and incontrollably foul that he should be "bound before the choir screen like a madman."

If this was really common practice, it bespeaks an ambivalent attitude which the church manifested toward the mad. On one hand, they were considered bestial, uncontrollable, loathsome to behold, stigmatized and, therefore, in need of salvation. On the other, they merited special charity, which the church, as the haven of love and the sanctuary of salvation, was bound to provide. The notion of charity has always been a forked one. Charity really means heavenly love, the opposite of earthly love or concupiscence. Yet charity also meant to people in the Middle Ages what it means today. It is a burdensome virtue which rewards only people who practice it upon their fellows who would normally evoke revulsion, hatred or, at least, rejection. The prosperous, the pleasant, the "natural" behavior is not an act of charity. Love of the poor, the demented, the insulting, the enemy—these are acts of charity which must be constantly preached because they are not normally practiced. When the church preaches charity toward the mad, as does the poet of *Piers Plowman*, it is indicating the natural repulsiveness of a segment of humanity which requires, for the sake of justice and virtue, an extraordinary sacrifice of instinctive behavior.

The doctors were obligated to treat the mad and to regard them with concern. The lawyers were charged with protecting the mad and their families and were obligated to be balanced in justice. The church was the haven of mercy and so would not simply damn its irrational children, but had to temper its condemnation with love. All of these "orders" of society were ambivalent in their attitudes toward the insane partly because their duties were so broad and their interests so complex. Yet, beside their literatures, grows another, the literature of courtly romance. The romance writers created their works for a narrow and quite clearly defined audience, and romance attitudes toward insanity were anything but ambivalent.

The insane heroes in courtly romance always take to

the woods, and their madness, like the environment to which it flees, is savage and terrifying. For the civilized audience addressed in courtly romances, any return to primitivism is mad. One courtly hero, Ywain, of *Ywain and Gawain*, is accused, because of his failure to fulfill his gentlemanly obligations and his consequent insanity and flight to the wilderness, of not being of "kynges blode." His failure to keep his vows is mad. He is sick in "will and herte" and he consigns himself to a lower order of being. He lives like an animal, so he is mad. He is mad, so he lives like an animal. The two statements are interchangeable in courtly circles. The maniac is the madman of the romances. The reasons are obvious. A violent and athletic figure is stranger, more dramatic. He offers us a flavor and an experience different from that of the meditative melancholic. He is action and plot and his plight seems more heroic because his behavior is more exaggerated. But we find an emphasis on fury and raging insanity in fiction that extends into the larger social realm as well.

In the literature of fiction, as in the literature of law, medicine and philosophy and even in folk sayings, the madman is not the melancholic but the more dramatic maniac. He is always the man who passes beyond the acceptable boundaries and is, thereafter, the outsider "out of his senses," "out of his mind," a stranger suffering from "alienatio," alienation because he is wild "wod" in English, "sauvage" in French. The fiction of the Middle Ages is the literature richest in terminology which it borrows from law, medicine and theology. The fiction reflects more than the bias of its authors; it reflects and perhaps contributes to a growing preoccupation with insanity which has not yet been satisfactorily explained. Yet from the fall of Rome to the fifteenth century, we begin to see an increasing interest in psychology. This bursts into full flower in the twelfth century and reaches a numerical zenith in the fifteenth. As modern readers, we are bound to wonder why the mad hero appears as a major figure in medieval literature for the first time in the twelfth century. Why was madness treated in such increasing detail from the twelfth century onward in medical and legal texts of England and the Continent?

The possible answers to these questions are many and varied and must, because of time and cultural differences, be speculative. First, the spoils of the Crusades included Aristotle's works and the manuscripts of the continuators of Galen. For the first time in the twelfth century, the learned of the church and students in the growing universities were treated to medical and philosophical works which had rested in Moslem libraries for centuries. Portions of these medical works exposed European students, clerics and physicians to healthy doses of anatomy, physiology and psychology and brain physiology which added to what they already knew about mania and melancholia. The scholasticism which grew out of this exposure and resulting devotion to Aristotle inspired a classifying urge which produced some of the greatest encyclopedias, which, in turn, made the materials of learning more concrete and available. The evaluation of and speculation upon science and philosophy led to a greater interest in the old "natures of things" which formed a natural link with the Augustinian examination of reason in the universe. One of these natures was, of course, human nature, seen now in terms of the interlinkage of "anima" and "animus" (of soul and spirit and mind) and of divine and human "logos" (reason). This influx of information which stimulated the intellect could not fail to stimulate the examination of the phenomenon of intellect.

In the literature of fiction, there was another new growth. The vernacular replaced Latin as the language of secular prose and poetry in increasing outbursts of nationalism. The product of this vernacular surge was a poetry and prose which broke with the old Latin tradition of the military hymn and the epic. The heroes of this literature were, in the first vernacular epics, mere embodiments of national and religious virtues, but, as romance, under the skillful hand of Chrétien de Troyes, became a major genre in medieval literature, the medieval audience was introduced to a new type of hero. This was the individualist who had to chart new territories, and fight, not in the mass phalanxes of the Romans or in the war bands of the pagans, but in hand-to-hand combat. His adversary became himself. Each battle, each foray into the wilderness was a test of virtues untried, for the hero of the romance faced his greatest ordeals in solitude. In this solitude, he became introverted. He examined the qualities of his own soul, the powers of his own reason, the conflicts between duty and the heart. The romance is a highly psychological genre. Chrétien de Troyes is the first romantic writer known to examine in detail the causes and complexities of a fictional hero's insanity.

Perhaps the increasing concern with insanity and its growing popularity as a literary motif arose in the sense of disorder loosed by the end of the Crusades. The holy wars abroad had served as an outlet for the energies of knighthood. European religion and philosophy advocated moderate behavior, called "measure," in all things.[22] Measured conduct seemed to the medieval mind, despite exceptions, the sine qua non of order. Only in a holy cause could immoderation be considered devotion and so the hero, an immoderate man by nature, found in the European moderation no outlet for his excessive bravery and devotion. In early works, to be heroic had automatically meant to be at one with society. Now increasing concern with individuals—individual language, individual writers and styles—meant increasing concern with personal identity which might lie beyond the bounds of society's demands and standards. In this search for identity within the social structure, the questing individual risked alienation. He was a stranger to order as status quo.

Since, in one manifestation, order was the operation of the divine mind on earth and, in another, it was that instrument which God gave to man in order to enable him to perceive His ordained order, a break with order was a break with reason. For the medieval mind all that is was meant to be part of order. Health was order of the humors, kingship was order of the government, faith was order of the soul. Chaos was pre-Christian evil; it pre-dated the creation itself and the medieval world embodies the devil, sin and destruction in chaos. A chaotic mind was ungodly. But madness terrified the populace then as it does today for reasons far from philosophical. It was strange, unpredictable, incomprehensible and threatening. For both philosopher and peasant the madman was, like the possessed, no longer a man. As the mad hero of the English fourteenth-century romance *Ywain and Gawain* cried out,

> I was a man, now I am none
> and all I lost for my folly.

# CHAPTER V

## Insanity in the Twentieth Century

In this conversation across the gulf of eight centuries, the dead have described madness in the Middle Ages. If the distance of time affords us complacence, the words of the living often destroy the illusion of progress. The subject of this chapter is insanity in the twentieth century and in America in particular.* This combination of time and nation provides the greatest possible contrast to medieval European attitudes toward insanity. Certainly modern readers expect to find in the United States of the 1970's the most dramatic break with the past. Some of the vital differences and similarities between madness in our own age and madness in the Middle Ages are best exposed by a glance at the medical, legal and popular concepts of insanity in the twentieth century. The results are often startling.

Perhaps the major difference between medieval and modern concepts of insanity is that medieval men knew what insanity was and we of the modern era do not. That is, medieval lawyers, doctors and theologians were certain of the symptoms and significance of insanity, however much they might define it according to their specialized

* The purpose of this chapter is not to advance modern law or psychiatry, but to propose some theoretical and deliberately idiosyncratic views of social history. For this reason the materials consulted are not intended to be comprehensive. If the reasons for my choice of particular texts are clear to the reader, that will be sufficient justification for their use in the service of stimulating further speculation about the origins of modern legal, philosophical and medical definitions and treatments of insanity.

interests and diagnose it in terms of behavioral signs. In the last decade, most legal treatises and psychiatric texts have reflected doubt about the meaning of the word "insane" and about the borderline between sanity and insanity. This is apparent in a current medical statement about a disease recognized as a form of insanity. "There are no objective criteria today for the diagnosis of schizophrenia."[1] It is further confirmed by a major legal paper, published in 1967, which affirms that "it is now apparent that a precise definition of insanity is impossible."[2]

Why was it possible to define insanity in the Middle Ages when it is so difficult to do so in the twentieth century? A very loose hypothetical definition of insanity evokes a series of answers to the question. Insanity is and was abnormal or asocial behavior pushed to unacceptable extremes. A prescribed sense of order, typical of medieval patterns of thought and analysis, simplified the observation of deviation from right or rational behavior. Aristotelian classification, increasingly popular from the twelfth century onward, promoted ease, if some variety, of definition in a society less tolerant and socially variable than our own. From the nineteenth century to the present, the phenomenon of "atomization" has affected every area of social life. The modern world with its rich variety of alternatives—religious, social, economic and philosophical—has extended the boundaries of normal behavior. The result has been increased flexibility and increased confusion, manifest in an unwillingness and even an inability to say what is rational or irrational, sane or insane.

Unwilling or unable, our physicians and lawyers are still forced to define insanity in order to prescribe and to judge. An unwieldy body of literature is the result, but the literature and its effects upon the insane in the modern world demand some detailed examination. Medicine and law have become the standards by means of which the fate of the insane is determined. Insanity in the modern world is still treated as a disease. Though modern psychiatrists complain that the language in which insanity is described is fallaciously derived from law, the medical literature on the subject is far more voluminous than the letters of the law. Psychiatry seems to precede forensic psychiatry and, for this reason, the terminology, symptomatology, etiology and therapy prescribed by the doctors must precede any understanding of legal and social attitudes toward insanity as disease.

The Salernitan documents provide the modern reader with a clear idea of the diagnoses and treatments of insanity which were standard to the teaching of medicine in medieval Europe. Although the medical literature on insanity has grown to mammoth proportions since that time, we are fortunate to be able to consult another standard. The *Comprehensive Textbook of Psychiatry*, edited by Alfred M. Freedman and Harold I. Kaplan, is widely used in American medical schools. Its definitions and treatments are fundamental to psychiatric training. It can serve as a modern Salernitan collection because it includes the modern and widely acceptable criteria, excellent for comparison and contrast with the medieval medical texts on insanity. In the sections on nomenclature and definition, this text avoids narrow and eccentric interests by drawing upon two universally recognized sources. These are the American Psychiatric Association's *Diagnostic and Statistical Manual* of mental disorders and the World Health Organization's international list of the causes of death, first authorized in 1853 and again in 1900.[3] The APA manual is numbered and keyed to match the WHO list. APA materials on mental disorder are more detailed, but the WHO list includes subcategories and variations of mental disease not commonly found in America. Despite the various objections to both lists, physicians are grateful for a convenient and general standard of classification from which they work.

One of the major problems in classifying and treating insanity today is terminology. In modern psychiatry the determination of insanity in a patient is inextricable from the name which is given the "disease" from which he suffers. The terms "insanity" and "derangement" no longer satisfy physicians. To be judged insane, a person must suffer from a condition with a name which means "insane." Even the closest modern approximation to a general term for insanity, the nineteenth-century "dementia praecox" (which refers to all forms of schizophrenia), is slowly falling into disuse. The commonest distinction between types of psychogenic diseases today is that between the less estranging and crippling neurosis and the more bizarre and alien psychosis. Yet, current psychiatry is discovering breakdowns even in the separations between less severe disturbances in neurosis and acute disorders in psychosis. The result is increasing discussion of "borderline states" between what medieval men would have called sanity and insanity and we, more hesitantly, call neurosis and psychosis.

Despite the proliferation of names for insanity or psychosis, modern psychiatry accepts certain diseases as psychoses. The major distinction it makes is one between psycho-biological psychosis which originates in permanent or temporary impairment of brain tissue, and psychogenic psychoses for which no totally physical origin has yet been securely identified. Most true insanity today is considered psychogenic and usually belongs to one of three large categories: schizophrenia of various types, paranoia of various types and acute manic-depression of various types, sometimes principally manic and sometimes principally depressive.

In general, the term "psychosis," applicable to each of these diseases or disorders, is used for "those types of mental disorders characterized by pervasive and profound alterations of mood, disorganization of thinking, and an associated withdrawal from the real world into a world of highly personalized preoccupations."[4] Even this seemingly innocent statement is a subject for debate. In the last two decades R. D. Laing, among others, has questioned the right of anyone but the patient to decide what reality is. Laing has proposed the notion of "separate realities" valid for each individual and incontrovertible by another whose reality sense, because his reality itself, is different from anyone else's. In an attempt to delimit psychosis in behavioral terms, Karl Menninger divided psychoses into "five classical categories." These are: a state of extreme despondency and guilt; an erratic excitement of both mood and motor functions; autistic behavior including irrelevancy, regression and bizarre thought patterns; "delusional preoccupation with one or several themes," such as suspicion, resentment, grandiosity, irascibility, etc.; disoriented states marked by confusion, delirious behavior, amnesia, hallucinations, etc.[5]

Of course, anyone may be temporarily preoccupied with suspicion or irascible, guilty or regressive without being considered psychotic by a physician. Furthermore, elements or traits mentioned in Menninger's list are frequently present in many neuroses. Conversely, many neuroses have not responded to treatment traditionally successful in such cases. All of these factors add to the general confusion and have made diagnosis of insanity or determination of normal behavior increasingly difficult. Despite all the skepticism and the hairline refinement of terminology, however, certain hard-core diagnoses and definitions of diseases considered forms of the forbidden disease physicians are loath to call "insanity," survive and bear marked resemblances to medieval forms of madness.

The disorder or disease most commonly attached to patients in mental hospitals is schizophrenia. Its forms are so varied that each of them may be diagnosed as a separate disease, a habit which was characteristic of the Middle Ages. There is hebephrenic or laughing schizophrenia, catatonic or stuporous schizophrenia, hyperactive catatonic schizophrenia and paranoid schizophrenia, characterized by delusions of either persecution or grandeur. In

any case, few physicians would hesitate to call true
schizophrenia a psychosis. The term itself means a severe
fragmentation of the thought process. The name was first
derived by Eugen Bleuler in the nineteenth century and
means "split mind." Bleuler identified three types of disturbances which formed the schizophrenic complex as:
disturbances of association, of affect and of activity. Other
psychiatrists have proposed further identifying criteria,
such as complete loss of contact with reality, the presence
of delusions and hallucinations, the loss of ego boundaries.

Characteristically, the schizophrenic withdraws from
others, speaks in symbols, is physically and emotionally
hypersensitive, has an alien perception of situations and
experiences, may be incoherent or mute and has a fragmented thought process. Although Soranus recognized
both extreme delusions of grandeur and stuporous states
as early as the second century, the disease of schizophrenia was not defined in the Middle Ages. This is true only
because neither classical nor medieval medicine conceived
of a process of splitting. The symptoms were recognized,
but they were never assigned a single name. Sometimes
the complex of symptoms was called a mania, sometimes
a melancholia, sometimes a form of possession. Yet, if a
single descriptive term did not exist, the symptoms of the
disease did and they were articulated by doctors and poets
alike.

Bizarre, delusional and regressive states are obvious in
Paul of Aegina's description of those who think they are
"brute animals and imitate their cries." References to
paranoid delusions of grandeur appear in his descriptions
of "those who think they are impelled by higher powers,
and foretell what is to come as if under divine influence;
and these are, therefore, properly called demoniacs or possessed persons." Delusions of persecution beset Aretaeus'
people who are "suspicious of poisoning or flee to the
desert from misanthropy."[6] The romances of the Middle
Ages are rich with heroes whose catatonia is manifest in

their lovesick refusals to eat and sleep, in their amnesia, in their blank mute stares. If love melancholy was the medical name for the disease during the Middle Ages, would catatonic schizophrenia or involutional depressive psychosis be the modern name for the disease? If obedience combined with derangement is a current complex in the behavior of catatonics, what would our psychiatrists call the disorder of the canine melancholics described in the Salernitan collection? They were those lycanthropes who were "affected with pugnaciousness, leaping and amentia. Sometimes this is combined with obedience, just as we see in the nature of dogs."[7] All the evidence points to the conclusion that the disease we call schizophrenia was recognized during the Middle Ages, but that it lacked a separate name.

This was not the case in the history of the manic-depressive syndrome. In its cyclical form, manic depression was recognized by Aretaeus the Cappadocian in the second century. Even modern historians who sometimes begrudge the earlier doctors their contributions to modern psychiatry cannot ignore Aretaeus' observation that "melancholy is the commencement and a part of mania. For in those who are mad, the understanding is turned sometimes to anger and sometimes to joy." The most startling fact about mania, melancholia and the manic-depressive syndrome is that the understanding of these conditions has not changed radically since the days of Homer, Hippocrates or Galen. Each of these disorders is still diagnosed largely by behavioral symptoms which are conceived of as clear and easily recognizable. The maniac is agitated, talkative, irritable and "elated," given to both physical and intellectual hyperactivity. The melancholic and the depressive are both exactly opposite from the maniac. They are mentally and physically hypoactive, sometimes anxious and fearful to the point of agitation.[8] The manic-depressive swings from mania to depression.

Although the form of depression known as involutional

psychosis is considered chronic and causes progressive deterioration, the manic-depressive condition is not generally considered either chronic or progressive. It is supposed to be subject to recurrences and remissions. Emil Kraepelin, the great modern pioneer in identifying this syndrome, was convinced, as Aretaeus had been, that acute mania and acute depression "only represent manifestations of a single morbid process." Aretaeus had said that this disease was different from a "confirmed madness [since it was] prone to imperfect intermission [and could] by some incidental heat of passion suffer a relapse." Kraepelin's conclusions were the same. Modern psychiatrists have recognized not only that the manic-depressive syndrome is a "folie circulaire," as a nineteenth-century Frenchman called it, but also that the manic-depressive syndrome as well as the psychotic depression usually follows upon the heels of some realistic cause. That cause could be either physiological or circumstantial.

## ETIOLOGY

A superficial glance at psychiatry today indicates that the concepts of the causes or origins of mental disease have changed radically since the Middle Ages. Yet comparisons of medieval and modern lists of possible etiologies of insanity suggest that in many cases we are following old routes in new vehicles. In the twelfth century Bartholomew of England listed as possible causes of madness: "passions of the soul . . . business, great thoughts, sorrow, too great study, dread, the biting of a mad dog or venomous beast, melancholy meats, drink of strong wine." In the thirteenth century, Arnold of Villanova suggested among the "interior causes of madness" passions of the soul such as "anger, sudden terror, hectic fever, too much fasting, insomnia and retention" of various types of blood which produced toxic states. Other classical and medieval physicians believed that seasons, climate, temperament and physiology (dictated by the astrological sign under which a person was born) were major factors in determining mental health or illness. In the twentieth century, psychiatrists have wondered if insanity is genetic or acquired, whether metabolic, electrical, hormonal, viral, biochemical, emotional or somatotypic.

Twentieth-century etiologies fall into the exterior or environmental and the interior or emotional and physiologic categories. In fact, the major argument about the etiology of insanity in the twentieth century has been the nature-nurture debate, which remains unsettled. The natural causes of psychosis are physical and genetic and they do include elements like metabolic rate, viral disease, hormone balance and electrical disturbances which were not understood in the Middle Ages. The modern nurture theory focuses upon environmental causes such as early emotional experience, later emotional trauma and unavoidable circumstances ranging from sibling rivalry to industrialization and from uprooting to war. Despite the vast differences between medieval and modern etiologies, the psychiatric evaluation of causes of insanity in the Middle Ages bears some remarkable resemblances to that in the twentieth century, in both specific and general cases.

In the case of involutional psychotic reactions, for example, the American Psychiatric Association's *Manual* says that individuals prone to the condition are "characterized by chronic, excessive, or obsessive concern with adherence to standards of conscience or of conformity. They may be overinhibited or overconscientious, and may have an inordinate capacity for work." These are certainly Bartholomew's men full of "business, great thoughts, sorrow, and dread" who go mad. The involutional melancholic appears as the compulsive mad knight of the medieval romance who is overcome by guilt because he has transgressed and betrayed the social ideal, or as the scholar who is a child of Saturn. Paul E. Huston notes that obsession with work and the sudden loss of the love object may both be contributing factors in producing an involutional psychotic depression.[9] His causes coincide with the medieval warnings that overwork can end in insanity and that loss of love and the consequent damming up of the sperm and/or menses both lead to madness.

Some of the closest parallels between medieval and modern etiology appear in the most unlikely areas. Medieval people believed in the predominance of the stars and planets in determining their physiques and psyches. Modern psychiatry has presumably abandoned this theory, yet, today, a number of psychiatrists and physiologists are working with findings that metabolism and physical qualities affect the psycho-biological constitution of a patient. Some physicians find that significant variations in the physiology of fetuses can be traced to the nutrition of the mother and that the diet she eats is often dependent on the time of year. Diet has even been cited as a factor in psychosis. Vitamin E therapy has been proposed as one cure for schizophrenia, and tryptophane, an essential amino acid, has been used in the treatment of depression.

Physiologic constitution has also been correlated with psychological constitution. The Middle Ages was not alone in believing that physical type and psyche were inextricable from one another. As late as 1921, "Kretschmer elevated these notions to a scientific study" in his assertions that there is a "pyknic manic-depressive type." One author asserts that there is a manic-depressive type of personality predisposed and, therefore, especially vulnerable to this disease. He observes that there are changes in "the metabolism of the adrenal steroids . . . in depression" as well as some changes in "electrolyte, water, and carbohydrate metabolism."[10] In schizophrenia, especially, physicians are prone to look for physical causes. Some have found abnormal constituents in the serum which they feel may cause a form of cerebral intoxication. An alternative theory is that the disease is caused by an enzyme defect in the central nervous system or a deficiency of a certain neurohumor, serotonin.

The medieval world was unacquainted with serotonin, carbohydrates, electrolytes and metabolic processes, but the more general concepts of predisposition, seasonal changes, the importance of diet and the interdependence of psyche and soma are the gross content of our modern discoveries. These ideas, expressed in other terms, were certainly familiar to medieval physicians. If they cured a disease by accidentally supplying the correct dietary insufficiency, they were still curing by diet. If they believed that they could detect a type of person prone to melancholy, we are not yet able to prove that they were totally incorrect, whether we agree or disagree with their theories. We do agree that some people are more prone to psychotic reaction from emotional strain than others, but the question of etiology of insanity has not yet been fully answered and, for this reason, even comparisons are on uncertain ground.

## THERAPY

The origins of insanity are both abstruse and abstract, whether they are modern or medieval, and the parallels between mysterious abstractions are more difficult to perceive. This is not true of the overt acts of therapy. Reasons for administering a treatment may be theoretical indeed, but the treatments themselves are clear and easily comparable. The general categories of modern psychotherapy are psychosurgery, chemotherapy or psychopharmacology, electroshock therapy, and the various forms of nonphysical or psychic treatment including psychoanalysis, group therapy, music therapy, play therapy, etc. Each had its medieval counterpart.

To the layman the most barbarous of all these practices is psychosurgery. The general name psychosurgery includes a number of different brain operations, notably lobotomy and topectomy. Although the radical practice of severing the connections between the frontal cortex and the thalamus has decreased since the advent of tranquilizers, it did presumably reduce "the intensity of emotional charge imparted to abnormal ideation."[11] From the pre-Christian era through the Middle Ages, a form of psychosurgery called trepanning was practiced. A hole was drilled in the cranium of the patient so that noxious vapors which had risen to the brain or evil spirits which were trapped in the brain could find a route of egress. In cases of brain tumors or collection of fluids on the brain, the operation was successful and the relief it brought lent weight and proof to the continued faith in the efficacy of the practice.

Modern psychosurgery springs from theories different from those which prompted the practice in ancient Egypt and medieval Europe, yet the justification for cutting arises from the medieval belief in the localization of brain functions and in the controlling force of psychic pneuma. That electrical charge which psychosurgery is supposed to interrupt is the modern form of psychic pneuma. The belief that lobotomy alleviates depression and agitation by sectioning frontal lobes in a coronal plane is similar to the medieval theory that worries and agitation are located in the front ventricle or imagination.

As ancient as psychosurgery, but less repulsive to modern patients and physicians, is chemotherapy. Today the pharmacopoeia of psychiatry is infinitely more extensive than it was in the Middle Ages and every year new drugs are added to the list. For depression we have mood-elevating drugs and drugs intended to inhibit the "depressing enzymes." For agitation there are tranquilizers. The ancients had opiates for mania and red wine for melancholy, but they, like us, operated on the allopathic theory of the efficacy of opposites. Sedatives, the poppies and lettuces used by the Arabs, depressed mania. Stimulants, like wine, elevated depression. Equally useful for the same purposes were the purgatives medieval physicians prescribed for melancholics. Emetic and laxative herbs could presumably rid the patient of maniacal and melancholic humors respectively.

In the case of the melancholic, the physicians hoped to purge the patient of the noxious black bile in the form of feces. Quaint and inaccurate as their theory may seem, physicians today recognize that depressives commonly report feelings of being full to the bursting point of what they often call "foul corruption." Since flatulence was reported as a common symptom of the ancient and medieval hypochondriacal melancholia, we might question whether or not a literal belief that constipation was the cause was responsible for the administration of purgatives. Perhaps the literal treatment of a reported symptom was an effective therapy which might be useful today. In the midst of rational-sounding prescriptions, we read of the value of the horn of the stag or the heart of an eagle and a treasury of other remedies which seem merely superstitious.

Electroshock therapy is as ancient as chemotherapy and as superstitious in origin. There are Roman discourses on the benefits of shock transmitted by electrical fish and portraits of electrical fish exist in even earlier Egyptian tombs. Of course, the theory underlying the ancient use of shock therapy has nothing to do with our current concept that it interrupts abnormal electrical patterns characteristic of mental illness and that it destroys waves peculiar to certain types of psychosis. It was based upon the belief that one horror or pain put to flight another. Electroshock was but one of the forms used. Sudden blows, showers of icy water, sudden frights are all forms of shock which have been used for centuries among primitive tribes, sometimes to drive out devils. The American film *The Snakepit* repeated the old superstition that new terrors catapult the patient out of a paralyzing depression; observations reveal that the empirical successes might have once again confirmed the practice of a treatment which originated largely in magic.

Both shock and psychosurgery are therapeutic techniques which seem technologically advanced for the Middle Ages and, for that reason, surprising. Their very physical nature, however, seems appropriate to an era popularly associated with brutality and unsubtle physical manipulation. More indirect and psychic methods of treatment are those which seem peculiar to the psychiatric modes of the twentieth century, but these too flourished in the Middle Ages. Music therapy, still in use today, was carefully explained in Byzantine documents which prescribed the proper scale or mode for the proper psychosis. Cheerful or martial modes were employed for elevating the moods of melancholics and sweet, gentle modes were played to maniacs. In fact, the prescriptions of the Byzantines indicate that music therapy had been refined to a degree that certainly equals, if it does not surpass, our own knowledge of its maximal use.

Hydrotherapy, one of the commonest means of calming agitated patients in modern mental hospitals, is repeatedly recommended in medieval treatises. The medieval rationale was that water cooled and moistened the hot, dry maniac. Paul of Aegina urged that "those who are subject to melancholy from a primary affection of the brain are to be treated with frequent baths, and a wholesome, humid diet together with suitable exhilaration of the mind, without any other remedy . . ." Bernard of Gordon said that "if the disease comes from dryness, warm baths should be given to the patient . . ."

Those Arab physicians who seemed so devoted to chemotherapy were also the greatest experts in psychic cures. To Arabic medicine and its later European successors, the world owes much of its knowledge of occupational and milieu therapy. Arab doctors recommended diversions like hunting, riding or walking as antidotes to melancholy. They believed that the mentally unbalanced should be exposed to pleasant sights and gardens and removed from all trauma. The earliest hospitals for the insane, like Fez, were equipped with beautiful gardens and decorative fountains designed especially to calm the fears and divert the concerns of the inmates. A later follower of the Arabs, Bartholomew of England, recommended that men should be removed from all unpleasant sights, including paintings, lest they be "tarred with madness." Today the structured workshop and the controlled hospital environment are the principal instruments of "milieu therapy," which is an attempt to produce a setting hostile to the patient's disease and encouraging to his reason and health.

The most apparently modern modality of treatment is, of course, none of these, but psychotherapy of the verbal variety. It ranges from the classic Freudian analysis to transactional and group therapy. Neither classic analysis nor group discussion was a medieval therapeutic mode, but the use of the physician, philosopher and priest as standards of normality and conversational therapists was. Soranus had advocated that "one help in curing them is to let them understand the lessons of the philosophers if they like, because these often dissipate fear and madness and help to re-establish health." Bernard of Gordon said that the man should "be obedient to reason and be removed from false examination." So sophisticated were some forms of therapy that physicians occasionally followed Soranus' early mandate to "alternate agreement with the patient's fantasies with disagreements with them so that the patient won't be hardened in his fantasies." Reassurance, support, insistence on reason, the recognition and identification of fantasy and its distinction from reality were all in the catalogue of psychotherapeutic aids long before the invention of psychoanalysis.

Despite the fact that modern historians of psychiatry are sometimes loath to credit the Middle Ages with any contribution to the study and treatment of insanity, the

Salernitan documents and the great medieval encyclopedists give the lie to modern condescension. Medieval psychiatric theorists must be credited with a rather long list of contributions to modern medicine. Not the least of these is their interest in and preservation of early Greek, Roman and Byzantine theories, an interest because of which they are accused of mere decadent imitation. In fact, whenever these ancient theories were available to medieval physicians and therapists, they incorporated and advanced them, forming a remarkably eclectic and varied approach to the problems of diagnosis, symptomatology and treatment of insanity. Their observations were remarkably acute and the medieval physicians should not be called "the unenlightened waiting for the Renaissance," for the Renaissance adopted many of the medieval theories.

The Arab physicians made numerous original contributions to milieu therapy, psychopharmacology and the study of schizophrenia, especially in their explorations of lycanthropy. Later physicians like Bartholomew of England contributed greatly to the holistic approach largely responsible for the psychosomatic medicine of today. Moralists like St. Augustine and St. Thomas explored the tortuous routes of conscience and its relation to biological drives. Surgeons like Constantine the African advanced the knowledge of brain anatomy and the localization of cerebral functions. Whether we bless or curse them for it, encyclopedists like Isidore of Seville in the ninth century, Bartholomew of England in the twelfth and Arnold of Villanova and Vincent of Beauvais in the thirteenth, are partially responsible for the size and weight of modern medical books. Their works are still valuable as a repository of past knowledge. They testify to an unquenchable intellect and an unfailing curiosity about the nature of the world. This curiosity was not only untrammeled by religious faith, it was positively encouraged by it.

Although the medicine of the Middle Ages seems far removed from us, we are beginning to return to the medieval interest in physical cause. There is an ever-increasing tendency to turn away from complete acceptance that the environment is omnipotent. Hard upon the heels of this rejection of a totally social responsibility for insanity follows an absorption in the study of physical causes like electrolyte balance, hormonal balance, genetic predisposition. These concerns and the growing conviction that mind and body are more interdependent than we had ever guessed are attitudes the medieval doctors would have found most congenial. Certainly there are vast differences between the psychiatry of today with its emphasis on child rearing and its belief in the curative power of memory, and the psychiatry of the Middle Ages. We know the differences and are usually ignorant of the similarities. Our "primitive precursors" arrived at many of the same conclusions we have, but their reasons for reaching them were different from ours. From the present-minded point of view, we are bound to say that medieval physicians had the right ideas for the wrong reasons.

## PSYCHIATRY AND THE LAW

If the medicine of insanity seems to have undergone some changes, the law of insanity seems to have undergone practically none. Neither forensic psychiatry nor the new mental-hygiene laws have arrived at universally satisfactory solutions to the ancient problems facing the insane at law. The courts still ponder the old subjects of Roman and medieval law: the definition of insanity; the determination of the existence of insanity in a particular individual by means of diagnostic criteria and legal tests; the rights of the insane in civil and criminal actions and in the modern addition, the course of hospitalization. Although citizens are constantly being declared insane, are hospitalized or are acquitted on grounds of insanity, the law has not been able to discover a clear definition of insanity. The new New York State Mental Hygiene Law of

1973 rejects the term "insanity" and defines a phenomenon called "mental illness" as a preferable substitute for the word "insanity." This substitution is partially due to the efforts of the Group for the Advancement of Psychiatry, who urged that "anachronistic terminology" be dropped and that "insanity and lunacy should be replaced by mental illness."[12] Yet as Bruce Ennis and Loren Siegel in their handbook, *The Rights of Mental Patients,* point out, "No one knows, for sure, what 'mental illness' means or what causes it."[13] In law as in medicine the terminology has changed but the diseases have not, and the new terminology, developed in order to remove the stigma from insanity, often obscures definitions and blurs distinctions and degrees.

Despite all the contemporary statements that insanity cannot be defined, jurists must identify the condition in order to implement both criminal and civil laws. The first major legal definitions of insanity in the modern law come, as the psychiatrists have claimed, from the jurisdiction of criminal law. In this country insanity is determined by "tests." The first and oldest of these is the famous M'Naghten Rule, proposed by the English courts in 1843 and accepted by all but one of the United States until the early 1950's. According to the M'Naghten formula, a person is considered criminally insane when he or she is "labouring under such a defect of reason, from disease of the mind, as not to know the nature and quality of the act he was doing, or if he did know it, that he did not know that he was doing what was wrong."[14] Complete ignorance and inability to distinguish right from wrong are the criteria or tests for insanity under this rule. Derivation from the old Roman law of the Twelve Tables is patent.

A sole dissenting American state, New Hampshire, operated under the so-called Durham Decision from 1870 on. The single criterion for determining criminal insanity under the Durham Decision was that the criminal act committed be "the product of mental disease." The other states, which retained the M'Naghten rule until the 1950's, added other criteria to the want-of-knowledge test. Chief among these was the "irresistible impulse" test. A person not in control of himself, or incapable of exercising free will, was judged insane. By 1954, the District of Columbia Court of Appeals announced a "new rule for the District in the Durham Case." Although the rule was very similar to the original, it stimulated much theorizing about and questioning of the old insanity laws throughout the country. Perhaps the most important result was the American Law Institute's proposal of a new test which was adopted by most states by 1971, after it had been incorporated in the Model Penal Code. This test separated the defect-of-reason criterion from the body of the definition and considered it a discrete element. The rule now reads: "A person is not responsible for criminal conduct if at the time of such conduct, as a result of mental disease or defect, he lacks substantial capacity either to appreciate the criminality (or wrongfulness) of his conduct or to conform his conduct to the requirements of law."[15] "Mental incapacity" was thus added to "lack of reason" and "lack of knowledge of right and wrong."

In criminal law, a person who is defined as criminally insane is one who has committed what is legally defined as a crime either as a result of his insanity or during the course of a period of insanity. To be criminally insane he must either be suffering from an irresistible impulse which he is powerless to perceive and overcome or be unaware of his actions and their criminality by virtue of his mental condition. Anyone who is criminally insane is considered free of responsibility for acts which would be felonious if committed by a sane person. Legal historians have traced the concept of insanity as a "mitigating factor which exempts the accused from punishment"[16] to the thirteenth century and have asserted that the concept of insanity as a "disease" originated with the M'Naghten Rule.

Actually, the two ideas long predate the thirteenth century. Exculpation on grounds of insanity is as old as the Roman law which declared that the insane could not be held responsible for what they were doing and should not be punished for their acts since insanity itself was sufficient punishment. The classification of insanity as a disease is as old as Hippocrates and as new as the medieval adapters of his theories. Both saw mental illness, especially in its advanced state, as the opposite of health and inextricably tied to the illness of the whole body. Insanity or unhealth was either physical in origin or physical in effect. Even the term "irresistible impulse," so novel in American law, derives from canon law and a belief in compulsion, usually demonic in origin. The doctrine of free will can be traced from the philosophical treatise of St. Augustine and through Roman law. The man who lacked free will was under the domination of a powerful alien force and could not be held responsible for his crimes.

Of course, it is possible to be insane without being criminally insane. The Group for the Advancement of Psychiatry has justifiably complained that most of the definitions of insanity are based upon "anachronistic terminology chiefly derived from criminal law."[17] Criminal-law definitions of insanity may indeed be vague, but, in the area of civil law, there are vast lacunae. The civil laws both free the insane of burdens and deprive them of certain rights and privileges, but there are no clear-cut definitions of insanity in civil actions. Instead, the laws governing treatment of the insane are scattered throughout specialized branches of civil law such as the New York State Domestic Relations Law and the Mental Hygiene Law of the same state.* The New York State Domestic Relations

* The New York State Mental Hygiene Law has been selected because it is so recent and is, therefore, representative of the most enlightened official views of the state. New York State laws have been used, for comparison, in the areas of domestic relations and wills and guardianship.

Law of 1967 uses a number of terms to define what is known as mental incompetence, a condition which is synonymous with legal incompetence. Among its criteria are "want of understanding," "incapacity to understand" and "unsoundness of mind." The new Mental Hygiene Law of 1973 cites such criteria as "impairment of judgment," "inability to understand," and uses the term "mental illness." Mental illness is defined as "an affliction with a mental disease or mental condition which is manifested by a disorder or disturbance in behavior, feeling, thinking or judgment to such an extent that the person afflicted requires care and treatment."[18] The terminology is both vague and disputed. In 1958, the author of a paper on forensic psychiatry could say, "I will say there is neither such a thing as 'insanity' nor such a thing as 'mental disease.'"[19] Nevertheless, this nonexistent state or condition is a bar to marriage, the making of wills and the administration of property.

The New York State Domestic Relations Law contains provisions for consent and contract very similar to those in Roman law and the articles of St. Thomas on marriage. "Before a marriage can be annulled on grounds of lunacy or for want of understanding of one of the parties, it must be shown satisfactorily that such party was mentally incapable of understanding the nature, effect, and consequences of the marriage."[20] Such a want of understanding can also be a bar to marriage since the party incapable of understanding is also legally incompetent. Insanity contracted after marriage can, in modern as well as Roman law, be sufficient grounds for divorce under certain conditions. The insanity must be proved "permanent and incurable." The annulment or divorce must be sought after a five-year period of the continuous insanity of one spouse, and providing that the husband is not only willing to but also did make specific legal provisions for the support of his wife during her entire lifetime, even after his death. Annulment may also be granted if, immediately after marriage, a husband, upon the instant of discovering his wife's insanity, "ceases to cohabit with her." The correlations between the old Roman and the New York State laws governing insanity and marriage are close indeed. Unlike Roman law, however, New York State law protects from annulment on grounds of fraud the person who did not report his continuing insanity to his spouse before marriage. The law notes that an insane person is "incapable of fraud and deception."

The laws governing wills have become increasingly complex, but, substantially, the essential requirement, soundness of mind, has not changed since Roman law, where "soundness of mind, not soundness of body is required of a testator." This remains in force today, when it is entirely possible for the aggrieved party to contest the will of any person he can prove insane or irrational at the time of the drawing of his will. This fact is familiar to any newspaper reader. The less familiar parallel to Roman law is the requirement that the executors be competent, a state which, of course, includes sanity. Executors can, according to the laws of Estates, Powers and Trusts, be replaced if they are incapable of either willing or enforcing anyone else's will. The term "will" itself recalls the very ancient equation of will with reason and of Augustinian free will with the later medieval definitions of sanity. The witnesses testifying to any will are testifying not only to its contents, and to its author's identity, but also to his sanity, the fact that he has a will of his own and can, therefore, make a will. Anyone who has no will of his own is considered incompetent.

Under most state laws, a person must be proved incompetent before he can be deprived of his legal status. The declaration may be judicial and the proceedings vary from state to state. Either one physician and a judge or any person and a judge, or several persons, including physician and judge, or any of these combinations with a jury must prove the insane person "incapable of juridical action."

If he is found legally incompetent, the insane or any other incapable person is entitled to the protection of an agent who will act for him. These agents or guardians are obligated to protect the rights and properties of their charges and they may be appointed by a court or a will. However, husbands are considered legal guardians for their wives and parents legal guardians for their children. Guardians are prohibited from either misusing or taking profit from their guardianships.

The types of guardianship are highly specialized in a system as elaborate as the Roman establishment. A guardian for a minor or adult incompetent is called a "guardian ad litem." A guardian principally charged with protecting the goods and property of an incompetent is called a "conservator." A more general guardian who is responsible for protecting all of the legal rights of an incompetent person is called a "committee." Obviously, legal guardians cannot be appointed for the insane until they are declared legally insane, but unlike the guardians of Roman law, American guardians can be removed at any point that the incompetent is declared legally competent by a court, assisted by the testimony of medical experts. The temporary or permanent incompetence of the guardian, his abuse or misuse of his charge's rights or property, is now, as it was at Roman law, grounds for dismissal.

Both the assumed guardianship of a husband for his insane spouse and the special guardianship required for an insane person are specifically designed, as the laws point out, to prevent the insane person from becoming "a charge upon the state." This detail and special provision indicates some major differences between Roman and medieval and modern society. There is a clearly defined state instrument for care of the insane in the United States. Since there were no such institutions in Roman and medieval society, there was little danger of state liability for care. Furthermore, the Roman and the medieval extended families were large units with clearly defined hierarchies

which carried with them specified legal responsibilities.
The dissolution of the family and the replacement of some
of its private functions by state organizations and institutions has meant an increasingly complex system of desig-
nation of responsibility. In many functions, the state has
replaced the clan or the family. At the same time, modern
concern with the niceties of human sensibility and the
abuse of permanent power has led many modern societies
to eliminate the institution of permanent guardianship
which was typical of Roman law.

The laws governing marriage, wills, crime and guardians of the insane are as old as the complex codes of law.
They are treated in many of the same terms as those by
which they were described in Justinian's laws. The completely modern phenomenon which we ironically call
"medieval" is the mental hospital establishment, which has
come to carry with it an immense corpus of laws, treatments, rights and provisions. In fact, the mental hospital,
as we have seen, did not exist in the countries of medieval
Europe. In the Arab nations of the Middle Ages which
did provide special facilities for the insane, there was nothing of the complex state institution of today, merely hospitals like any others for the chronically ill. The modern
mental hospital did not begin to come into existence until
the sixteenth century, the height of the period of enlight-
enment. By the seventeenth century, Europe and England
were the proud possessors of what Foucault called the
"great judicial" establishments, the madhouses to which
one might be confined by the law.

Today, throughout the world, a gigantic complex of
governmental and private hospitals for the insane has created an establishment of madness. In the United States
the variety and number of hospitals and laws for admission
to and administration of them provide a composite biography of insanity in the twentieth century. The laws and
the hospitals themselves are as different as the localities
within which they function. For these reasons our case

histories and discussion will concentrate upon America and its state or governmental hospitals which now survive and operate under specific state laws that often determine the case history of the madman or psychotic in America.

To be admitted to a state hospital in this country, a prospective patient must consider the alternatives. There are many kinds of admission. The informal or voluntary admission is a process conducted by the patient at his own will and, presumably, entitles him to leave the hospital at any time. Minors, however, can be committed on a voluntary basis against their wills by a guardian or relative. The involuntary or formal admission is a process conducted by someone (other than the adult patient) who believes that the patient is sufficiently mentally ill to be "in need of care and treatment" (the New York State Mental Hygiene Law's current criterion of recognized need for admission to a mental hospital). The patient need not necessarily be considered dangerous. Prior to admission, the patient is presumably examined by the admitting physician or hospital director, who must concur in his findings with anyone admitting the patient.

Patients involuntarily admitted are not free to leave at their own wills without undergoing a formal examination. There are two types of involuntary admission procedures: the emergency and the non-emergency admission. Under the emergency admission procedures, the patient can be simply detained or even what we would call "arrested" and then detained by a mental facility. The emergency admission, although it specifies a limited period (this period varies enormously from state to state) during which the admittee must be examined and found mentally ill or else discharged, is a more immediate and sometimes more threatening procedure. It can be conducted by a layman, a community-health officer, a law officer, a doctor or a relative and requires no court sanction. Presenting symptoms can be as vague as "funny behavior." The non-emergency involuntary procedures of many states do require prior sanction or confirmation before admission, either by a court and some qualified psychiatric experts or by one of the two. In an admittedly polemic study, Bruce Ennis and Loren Siegel point out that, in England, 80 percent of the mental hospital admissions are voluntary, whereas, in the United States, the ratio is reversed. Let us follow the course of one voluntarily admitted mental patient to gain insight into the process of hospitalization.

Miss Bamber, whose mother, her last surviving relative, had just died, was a scholarship student at a large university in New York City. After her mother's death, she experienced persistent attacks of general fear. She was afraid to walk alone in the streets in midday. She was convinced that she would die an early and unnatural death, about which she dreamed in various forms—struck by a runaway driver, being pushed from her apartment window by a stranger. Because she had to take examinations on which the continuation of her scholarship depended, she tried to put aside her anxieties and concentrate upon preparation, but her irrational fears intruded upon her studies. However, she prepared as well as she could and went to take her examinations, which she completed. On her way home from the university, she thought she heard her name being called. She turned to look for a familiar face but did not see one in the rush-hour crowds. That night she woke screaming from a nightmare about being pushed into an open grave. She turned on the light to read in order to calm herself, but, in the middle of her reading, she heard her mother's voice calling her. After several days of auditory hallucinations, she became sufficiently alarmed to seek psychiatric aid at her university clinic. One day she did not keep her appointment with her therapist, who was concerned and called her apartment for the remainder of the day. Just before closing time at the clinic, he received a call from the city hospital's local psychiatric facility. Miss Bamber had signed herself in as a voluntary, informal admittee. She had referred the admitting psychiatrist to her therapist. After examining her, the admitting psychiatrist, in consultation with her therapist, agreed that she was "in need of care and treatment."

When she was signing herself in to the hospital, Miss Bamber, desperate for care and shelter and frightened by her hallucinations, was unaware that, as a standard part of admission, she had signed the usual series of waivers. These included a shock waiver—a legal document which waives the patient's right to refuse shock treatments, only in case the professional staff of the hospital considers her "incapable of making a rational decision" (the New York State Mental Hygiene Law's phrase for incompetent or insane) about the treatment "of which she was in need." Miss Bamber remained in the hospital and was given regular appointments with a therapist. After three weeks she received a notice from the director of the hospital that the staff deemed suitable and necessary a change of her status from voluntary to involuntary. She did not know and was too distraught to comprehend the appended provision that she was entitled to a court hearing in this case. A change in her status meant that the physicians considered her unable to make a rational decision "about her own care and treatment" and the optimal date of her discharge.

Several days later, while she was in her room, a nurse approached her, carrying a hypodermic needle. When she asked what it was for, she was told that it would "help her relax." She refused the injection and was forcibly restrained in a straitjacket and her physician was summoned. Considerably more passive, she asked what the hypodermic was for and what it contained. He told her that it contained sodium pentathol and that it was to help her sleep during a shock treatment which would make her better. She said that she did not want shock and, although the doctor was too tactful to tell her so, he was going to proceed with the treatment on the grounds that she was not able to make rational decisions about the care and treatment of which she was in need.

Two months later, Miss Bamber was released with fifty dollars and "suitable clothing" as the state construes the phrase. Among the articles returned to her she did not find a small sapphire ring left her by her mother and a watch which had been a high school graduation gift. These had been, legally, sold at the director's discretion to pay some of the expenses incurred by the patient.[21]

Miss Bamber was more fortunate than she might have been. The physicians could have performed psychosurgery against her will, for example, and, before the new Mental Hygiene Law of 1973, she could have been told to "work for her own sake" in a hospital kitchen, laundry or library or at a cleaning job for which the hospital did not pay her. Such enforced work, Ennis and Siegel point out, is a form of peonage which is unconstitutional and which, by the way, is never assigned to regular patients at non-mental hospitals. She might, on the other hand, have called in the Mental Health Information Services, a quite new legal association devoted to the care and civil rights of patients and now written into many mental-health laws as a reviewing committee on patient status and rights. Had she been hospitalized prior to the enforcement of the 1973 Mental Hygiene Law, she might have received treatment but then, again, the hospital might have acted in any entirely custodial capacity, since there was not any law, prior to 1973, which "obligated" the hospital to provide treatment. Indeed, in many states, such as New Hampshire as of 1973, state mental hospital facilities are under no obligation to provide care and treatment, may open patients' mail and may severely restrict all visitation rights —always, of course, on the grounds that these measures are in the therapeutic interests of a patient who is unfit to make such decisions. Some states have no laws requiring hospitals to inform patients of their rights or their change of status or even their transfer to another suitable facility, a procedure which is legal in almost every state. Some states still require a patient to work without pay. South Dakota, among other states, had no provision, as of 1973, for confidentiality of patient records. South Carolina can legally sterilize any patient whose insanity is deemed "hereditary." Virginia has no provision to restore the status of mental competence after a patient's release from the hospital, a provision New York State has written into its new laws. Even religious freedom is not necessarily stipulated for mental patients by many states, among them Wisconsin. Mississippi has no legal provisions for right to treatment, communication and visitation, civil rights, religious freedom, payment for work, notices of patients' rights, control of personal property, voluntary admission, right to a free lawyer, provision of adequate clothing on discharge, penalties against physicians or hospital staff for abuse of patients or their rights, or periodic review of patients' status and condition.[22]

As more moderate thinkers and legislators might point out, the lack of such legal provisions is by no means necessarily symptomatic of official viciousness or lack of humanity. It may arise from oversight, from overtrust, from lack of social or legal vision. What is horrifying is the list of abuses which can result from such oversights or omissions. Under the authority of an either careless or deliberately inhumane or even merely biased administrator, a Mississippi mental-health patient can be deprived of all property, incarcerated and held virtually incommunicado in a hospital in which he is denied the right to the comforts or practice of his religion. He can be kept in the hospital uninformed of his rights or condition without receiving any treatment for that condition. He can be beaten or oppressed in any number of ways by a hospital staff or physician not liable under any specific law for maltreatment. Finally, he can be released, at will, but with no funds or clothing. His record can be divulged at will by the hospital and he may thus continue to be deprived not only of the right to work, a constitutional right under federal law, but also of the right to vote, to administer property, to be legally married.

Indeed, perhaps the most serious question of all for mental patients has been that of civil rights. Unless a state law specifically provides for the restoration of civil rights or at least for the right to free legal counsel, an indigent patient (and indigents are the largest population of state mental hospitals) can remain in the status of second-class citizen for the rest of his life. Unless a precise provision is made for protection of patients' rights, hospitalization for mental illness can cancel these rights. The New York State Mental Hygiene Law (15.01) now has a provision that "notwithstanding any other provision of law, no person shall be deprived of any civil right, if in all other respects qualified and eligible, solely by reason of receipt of services for a mental disability nor shall the receipt of such services modify or vary any civil right of any person, including but not limited to civil service ranking and appointment, the right to register for and to vote at elections, or rights relating to the granting, forfeiture, or denial of a license, permit, privilege or benefit pursuant to any law."

We have seen how difficult the lot of the voluntary patient whose status is later deemed involuntary can be. Even more shocking is the situation in which the emergency involuntary admittee may find himself. Most states still make fairly flexible rules about initial emergency admission procedures, although, as we have noted, the period of retention under such a status without review is usually limited. In Oregon, for example, any patient admitted under the involuntary emergency procedure can be detained no more than forty-eight hours without being examined by two staff doctors who, on confirming the emergency, apply to the superintendent. The superintendent must either obtain a voluntary admission from the patient or apply to the courts for involuntary admission. Ohio, on the other hand, permits a detention period of sixty days following the allegation of any person that the admittee is dangerous, confirmed by the certificate of a doctor.[23]

Why and how is insanity observed by a hypothetical layman or apprehending officer? What can be some of the reasons for non-voluntary and non-voluntary emergency hospitalization? One clinical psychologist who was employed by a state mental hospital recently pointed out a perfectly sane-looking woman to a visitor. The woman had been committed by her son-in-law and daughter under an involuntary admission procedure. When he was asked what her illness was, after he had carried on a perfectly lucid and intelligent conversation with her, our psychologist replied, "She likes to talk to trees." "What are her other symptoms?" the visitor asked. "None," he replied, "except that she likes to talk to trees." This state has relatively poorly defined admission procedures. The law honors any person, armed with statements from two doctors alleging that the prospective patient has a "mental disorder," so that "for his own protection and that of others," he "requires care and treatment and is unwilling and unable to apply voluntarily therefor." The patient's behavior was unattractive or frightening to her relatives. Sane people don't talk to trees. This was an embarrassing situation and who knew what it might lead to? She was clearly irrational if she talked to trees and also refused to submit to hospitalization because of it. Often the arguments of the mental hospitals are, as Ennis, Siegel and others point out, circular. A patient who wants to be discharged must be irrational if he does not feel he needs further care and treatment and, if he is irrational, he is not sufficiently competent to be discharged. The psychologist felt that, from his point of view, much of the state hospitalization throughout the country was cosmetically motivated and custodially executed. That is, people were too often committed for behavior which relatives, law officers or ordinary laymen thought "strange," "scary," "not normal" or "disturbing" and were, after admission, merely fed and clothed. Some of these admissions were involuntary non-emergency procedures; some were emergency procedures.

Although a number of states do not have emergency procedures and many which do have stipulations that emergency admission procedures may be used for patients not considered "dangerous," many states include diagnosis of "dangerous" among the major reasons for emergency admission. Often the term "dangerous" is not defined. In the more scrupulous judicial procedures and the more progressive mental-hygiene laws, like that of Massachusetts for example, it is defined as "dangerous to others or to himself," which we may understand simply as homicidal or suicidal, but the thorn is that the danger, unless criminal insanity has been found, is frequently potential danger. In short, the diagnosis or treatment is preventive, a laudable aim in medicine of all kinds, but sometimes a treacherous practice. What is the effect of preventive hospitalization? How certain can even an experienced prophet be about future danger? In both the execution of such predictive care and the more civil libertarian rejection of it, fatal errors and serious injustices are committed. Lee Harvey Oswald was declared potentially dangerous by a high school counselor. He realized his potential. Other patients who have been preventively hospitalized on a concurrence of two doctors that they were potentially dangerous have been foolishly, wastefully and unfairly detained.

Was not only the provision for "need of care and treatment" but also the "potential danger" provision operating when, during the writing of this last chapter, a man named Petit secured a high wire between the two highest buildings in the world, the two towers of the World Trade Center in New York City, and proceeded to walk between them in the early hours of the day? He was observed carrying the tightrope walker's pole and skillfully threading his way back and forth across the wire. The police ordered him to descend, but he lay down on the rope midway between the buildings and refused. When he finally did come off the wire, the police were prepared to admit him involuntarily to Bellevue, City Hospital's ward for the mentally ill. The police persisted in their conviction that he should be hospitalized, despite the fact that the man was, by his own statement and those of others, an experienced tightrope walker who liked new challenge. He was finally released after he promised to give some charity performances for children. Was he dangerous? Yes. High-wire walking is a dangerous sport for the performer and, in this case, for any potential passers-by. Was he insane? Is every circus performer insane? Certainly his behavior was unorthodox, but such a response to it is more than vaguely reminiscent of the medieval church's epithet of "madman" for any heretic and the cry of "possessed" flung at Margery Kempe by those who refused to accept her response to a mystical experience as sane.

## SOCIAL ATTITUDES AND ANCIENT SURVIVALS

Perhaps the most instructive aspect of the two anecdotes of the tightrope walker and the woman who befriended trees is the social attitude they reveal. They lead us to the larger questions which lawyers and political philosophers are beginning to consider. The fiction of our day is also much concerned with both the real and the metaphorical meaning of insanity. In fact, although the terms "insanity" and "lunacy" are becoming unpopular in this country, the phenomena, the discussion of them and the figures of speech based upon them not only survive but continue to multiply. In cities, many observers report what appears to be a greater number of obviously insane people. Growing numbers of laymen commonly use the term "schizoid." "Schizy" is a common slang term. Paranoia seems, if we listen to ordinary conversation, to be as com-

mon as the cold. Some of the terms may be new but the
attitudes toward insanity, whether we call it psychosis or
madness, have changed little since the Middle Ages.

The medieval worship of reason is still in force. Our
highest praise for an argument or a course of action is that
it is rational. Our most serious diagnosis of the physical
condition of a patient is that he is "irrational," a term
which evokes sad and sage nods from the listener. The
most prevalent response to insanity is fear, because it "just
isn't natural" and people who are mad "don't act human."
They are unfamiliar and, worse, unpredictable. We even
deny the possibility of a real insane self, and say that, in
insanity, a person is not himself, harking back to the
priestly belief that a person is someone else when he is
insane. Who is he? Except for theologians concerned with
the incursions of the devil into the human mind, few people realize that the concept that an insane person is someone else is a direct outgrowth of the ancient idea that another power could dominate a man's mind from outside.
Historians point out the derivation of our word "obsessed"
from the religious ideas of "possession." Obsessional neuroses and psychoses are expressions of such total absorption in one subject that all other concerns are eradicated.
So it was supposed to have been for the demonically possessed whose minds were so rigidly ruled by a demonic
master that they were not "in control of themselves," an
expression we still use in both law and common parlance.

Recently a man murdered a number of coeds on Long
Island and, when he was apprehended and charged with
the crimes, he used as his defense a form of the insanity
plea so old that it seemed ingeniously new. He claimed
that he was in the power of the devil when he committed
those crimes and was, therefore, not in control of his actions. The court seriously entertained the case but finally
the scientific skepticism of our age prevailed and the defense was dismissed. The murderer was, in fact, only taking advantage of the current recrudescence of demonology

in our country, but he had tapped an interesting historical connection between innocence of guilt, loss of free will, temporary insanity and possession by the devil, a complex of ideas which still flourishes in more minds than we like to admit. The folk expressions that we are "full of the devil" or in a "diabolic rage" or "bedeviled" or looking "haunted" merely mask vague concepts about the loss and invasion of the self and self-control.

For the more scientifically oriented, the most convenient term for insanity is "mental illness," the much disputed phenomenon of our age. It too reflects the medieval beliefs in wholeness and health. The continuing belief in insanity as a disease, parallel to physical disease, has spurred much modern research into physiological origins of mental states and even a survival, legalized by some states, of the belief that insanity may be hereditary. Oddly enough, we have abandoned popular belief in the direct inheritance of physical diseases, but many of our laws, like the sterilization law, are still designed to protect potential offspring from the ancient taint of hereditary insanity, a genetic legacy of which we are far from certain.

Classical and medieval theories of medicine and philosophy also survive in the belief in balance. It seems unlikely that we shall ever dispense with the concept that balance is vital to life. A balance of diet, a balance of hormones, a balance of fluids and electrolytes may be certifiably essential, yet the expression "he is unbalanced" still means exclusively: he is not sane. It grows out of the concept of the four elements which is transferable to the four humors and the four temperaments and, finally, in a moral sense, to the control of the passions. Throughout history, balance has been considered a divine attribute and a precept for human behavior. The Greeks constructed their buildings according to an ideal of balance and proportion. For the Romans, stoic control of the passions was not only a moral axiom, but, presumably, a physical necessity. Any overindulgence could tip the scale of balance.

To this day we prohibit the fullest exercise of the emotions and speak in nearly physical terms of being "crazed with grief," dominated by a "maniacal rage," seized with "maniacal laughter," "insane with fear" and "mad with desire." The stoical concept of control of the emotions became, under the Christian aegis, the theological system of the deadly sins. Those whom the gods would destroy, they first drive mad, became those whom the devil would destroy are first ensnared by deadly sins. In the modern world the cast of sin has been reshaped. The sins are the same but we do not regard them as sins. We regard them again, as the Romans and Greeks once did, as either willful abandonments of self-control, forms of deliberate self-indulgence or the unwilling loss of control through some form of illness. Even the law, in its most abbreviated formulae, preserves the philosophy of proportions in its exculpation of anyone who commits a crime with the "balance of his mind disturbed."

The distribution of our various attitudes toward the insane comes from all of the spheres of the medieval world and carries with it all of the ancient biases and charities. The formulae of the church urged mere pity and comfort toward the mad while simultaneously ascribing tainted morality and evil to a man who is in the grips of a certainly ungodlike and therefore unnatural, even occasionally demonic, force. This ambivalence survives in our expressions. "What possessed him?" we ask. He was suffering from an "irresistible impulse," our laws, derived from canon law, tell us. We must offer him charity and shelter, our word "asylum" reminds us. He has lost the godlike quality, our word "irrational" tells us. From the medical legacy we inherit the concept of balance, "ill" or "strange humor," being "out of one's senses," being "impaired in our judgment," being "diseased" or unhealthy. From the lawyers, we inherit the terms "out of control," "incapable of action," "incompetent." From the theologians and from medieval hierarchical society which so often expressed itself in fiction, we retain the terms "inhuman," "savage," "unnatural," "wild man."

Admittedly, these are "merely expressions" and most modern men believe that expressions long survive their origins and the early beliefs which prompted the old phrases. But in certain survivals, although the conscious awareness of the original meaning has been lost, some of the unconscious beliefs which lie buried help to preserve the underground survival of the ancient ideas. What can we mean when we say that a man is "beside himself," if we do not suggest that the soul may go out of the body as medieval men thought it could? What do we mean when we say that a man has "lost his senses," unless we still believe that the senses lie in the interior world at the center of full health, as the Arabs said they did? What do we mean by "crazed with grief," except that what Bartholomew called "interior passions" could cause madness? What do we mean by "seizures of emotion," unless we are still convinced that emotions can come from some outside force, as the devil could "compel" a man to do something uncharacteristic? What do we mean by "lunatic," unless we still believe in the psychic state provoked to unpredictable and uncontrollable cyclic episodes of madness by the waxing and waning of the moon? Workers in mental-health facilities have often observed that, on nights when the full moon is shining, patients exhibit more bizarre symptoms, more extreme manifestations of their usual symptoms. We have yet to discover if the moon, which now seems to control so many cycles besides those of the tides, can, in fact, influence the human mind. Perhaps the patients are themselves instinctively responding to old myths. Perhaps the observers, because they are unconsciously operating under the force of old beliefs, tend to influence the behavior of their patients, who sometimes are reportedly hidden from the view of the moon and unaware of its phase.

Just as the names for causes and symptoms of insanity

survive in the minds of the sane, so they survive in names the insane call their own delusions or hallucinations. In schizophrenia, for example, the suffering patient not infrequently sees himself as an object, though not usually the cracked pot of the ancients, a term which still survives in the minds of those who often call the insane "crackpots." Yet the delusions of grandeur of the paranoid personality still fix on Christ as a delusionary model, as the author of *The Three Christs of Ypsilanti* pointed out. Succeeding historical figures are added with each age and the most familiar of these is Napoleon, but every martyred and powerful figure is meat for delusion, which may be flexible, inventive, up to date. May not former President Nixon be a future delusionary model for the paranoid personality who seeks his identity with the great, the beleaguered and the misunderstood?

Modern technology provides particularly dramatic "influencing machines."[24] An all-powerful technology lends itself with peculiar elegance to the delusionary system. Lynn White mentions the profound terror caused by the invention of the so-called perpetual-motion machines, which formed perfect objects of delusion for medieval psychoses after the thirteenth-century theories about them. It would naturally have been impossible for a medieval psychotic to have created the fantasy of a young man in the 1960's who carried a broken transistor radio with him and could not talk until he pressed the "on" button or stop speaking until he pressed the "off" button. Reality and fantasy now merge in technology. Big Brother may, in fact, be watching us on a closed-circuit supermarket television or listening to us through a bugging device. The person who suspects that his telephone is being tapped can no longer be dismissed as paranoid.

Despite all the changes in technology and the alteration of reality, the symptoms of mental illness remain the same. The seriously depressed still experience a "desire for solitude" and what modern and medieval psychiatrists called "feelings of withdrawal, fear and suspicion." Paranoid schizophrenics, like the medieval possessed, hear voices and feel that they are being told to do things they do not wish to do. On the other hand, we must face the possibility that we believe the past even while we are denying its validity, and that, believing it, we seek to confirm it, sometimes by means of our new God, science. Saddest of all is the possibility that the modern era, which cherishes the conviction that its science and its social attitudes have surpassed and even disproved those of the "positively medieval" world, has not progressed very far. The most dramatic alternatives are that they were brilliant or we are stupid.

The underlying social or popular attitudes toward madness, too, belie the concept of a revolutionary or modern age. Presumably enlightened people shrink at the suggestion that the mad are to be regarded with any feelings other than sympathy and concern, but one need only observe the speech and affects of a so-called normal man whose instinctive response is often one of contempt-masking fear. We admire competence and the insane are legally "incompetent." We depend upon reason and the insane are irrational. We pursue health and the insane are unhealthy. Although we try to consider insane behavior as alternative to our own, we in fact consider it a flawed form of our own. We deny increasingly the existence of a phenomenon called "normality," yet we call the behavior of the schizophrenic "abnormal," thereby admitting the closet survival of an ideal not far different from the medieval ideas of order and a recognizable standard of right, virtuous behavior. We still say, "His mind isn't right," revealing the fact that we believe there is a right and a wrong mind. Today the insane are still "the other," little different from the alienated ones, as people once called those who were treated like aliens because they inhabited another and a strange "country of the mind." So too the insane regard their adversaries, those who do not

think the way they think, those who are forever insisting
that their own mode of thought is to be emulated because
it is a standard. This is a situation not peculiar to insanity.
The different have always been regarded with suspicion
and fear and the resulting dislike which springs from the
assault of negative and threatening emotions. We may ex-
cise the words "insane" and "alienist" and "lunatic asylum"
from our vocabularies, but it is unlikely that we can ever
eradicate the feelings and the history of feelings they embody. Nor am I suggesting that we should; however, we
should be aware of the fact that we still feel that the insane are aliens, that they are in some way guilty and
therefore deserving of insanity and that they represent that
most taboo of all states—chaos.

Insanity is, after all, now called, in the liberal tongue, a
"mental disorder," a term which evokes images of mental
order. Yet psychiatrists recognize a very clear and psychological order in the thought processes of various forms
of mental disorder. Although the concept of order is older
than Christianity, its most articulate and influential proponents in the modern world are still the descendants of
the Judeo-Christian, rather than the Greek, philosophies
of cosmology. The principal proof of the existence of God
has been, for the last seven centuries, order which descends to man and is, as theologians have noted, epito-
mized in the reason, synonymous with order, which
descends from God to man. The principal metaphor for
the existence of the devil is chaos and disorder, synonymous with hell, darkness and suffering.

Mental patients confined to an institution which they
find threatening, frightening or unpleasant often speak of
it in these same words used by the sane to describe insanity. It is chaos. It is a place ruled by those who seek
to impose order of their own on a populace incomprehensible to them. It is a place for the habitation of the
damned. In fact, mental patients frequently describe the
hospital in terms the medieval man would have under-

stood. "It is hell," they say, or "We are in hell." Each ward which progresses further toward release is a step toward purgatory, which is reached by entering the outside world. For others, the hospital seems a place of punishment, staffed by wardens, and they feel that they are in prison. For still another portion of the population, the hospital is a haven from the threatening world and a home in which they are protected from themselves and others. Many of these people prefer the safety of a sheltered world in which they do not have to greet the strains and horrors of the unpredictable and sometimes solitary life of the "outside." In these cases, they are happy to live in what we are horrified, and they are delighted, to call an "asylum."

The philosophy which supposedly underlies the maintenance of closed wards and solitary rooms today is identical to the rationale for the chaining or sequestering of the insane in the Middle Ages. In Hannah Green's account of her hospitalization, she describes a particularly acute attack "from" her sickness during which she was helped by an understanding hospital staff member. "Is the word fear?" she asked. "No—not fear—anger." And then, looking at Deborah again: "An anger you cannot control." After a pause she said, "Come on, we'll try seclusion until you can take care of yourself." Later her doctor says, "You are afraid of your power and that you cannot control it." She explains to her patient, "It is why you need a hospital. You are in a hospital and you do not need to fear the terrible forces that seem to have been opened in you." In Rome and later medieval Europe the mad were prescribed containment and even mechanical restraints, not for punishment, but so that they could protect themselves and others from harm.

The advent of the system of mental hospitals, licensed and controlled by states and governments, is, perhaps, the only completely novel contribution of modern society. Therapy of every kind now used in a higher technological form is, of course, not new. The discovery of disease is not new. Systems of laws protecting the rights of the insane in the larger society out of which they come are not new, but a social provision for care of both rich and poor insane is new in the West. The economic determinant in the quality and easy availability of psychiatric and physical care is still a realistic factor, but even the force of economics is mitigated by current mental-hygiene facilities in the more comprehensive state systems.

That governments have an obligation to care for the insane and the indigent is an idea as old as the fourteenth century. The vast and general network of hospitals of different types is a distinctly twentieth-century phenomenon. Even more recent is the advent of a unified-services program for mental-health care in a number of states. This plan attempts to eliminate redundancy and to provide a broad range of types of service to the mentally ill by utilizing, as effectively as possible, all the mental-health facilities available to the public. The establishment of such a system, designed to help both society at large and the insane in particular, seems beneficial, but we should not ignore the negative consequences of systematized confinement. Modern America, like Europe, no longer sends its mad away on ships; it no longer exiles them to the forest or drives them away from the towns or beats them in the streets or meets them wandering in cold and hungry crowds begging on corners and highways; but it has a "place" for them. Nevertheless, the very existence of such a place in which they can be securely confined means a deprivation of freedom. Without the existence of such a well-organized institution as the mental hospital or the mental-hygiene complex, the organized implementation of shock therapy, drug therapy, psychosurgery and sterilization would be infinitely more difficult. The organization of concerned and consistent treatment for acute cases, as well as the institutionalized cruelty practiced occasionally by exasperated and frightened attendants, would also be impossible. The insane man in the Middle Ages could be victimized by the townspeople, but the victimization, like the care, was disorganized. Greater neglect meant greater freedom even if that freedom was the liberty of neglect. Social progress is the history of institutionalized interference.

Although citizens are now exerting pressure on mental hospitals to keep patients out of the community, some states, notably California, concluded in the 1960's that hospitalization itself perpetuated alienation. The longer a patient was separated from society, the advocates of early release argued, the more involuted grew his desocialization. In an attempt to remedy the hospital virus of the psychiatric ward, California advocated and practiced early release of mental patients and their gradual reintegration into a normal life through outpatient care.* Patients were re-placed into their natural, though somewhat more carefully structured environments. Centuries earlier this philosophy was tried in Gheel, Belgium, where it is still in force. There patients have been spared hospitalization by being cared for in special family environments which are constructed to receive and treat the mentally ill in circumstances which simulate as closely as possible the freedom and warmth of real families. The result, however, has been the creation of a village of the insane. Everyone knows it is a village of madmen, but, because of its social structure, the sane caretakers are frequently visibly indistinguishable from their insane patients.

In fact, Gheel is the real-life model of an old medieval metaphor which is becoming increasingly popular in modern fiction. This is the metaphor of the world as a madhouse. Its most notable representation in modern fiction

---

* This practice is changing because of community fear. One Long Island community has instituted an ordinance which, in effect, prohibits former mental patients from taking up residence.

is Ken Kesey's *One Flew over the Cuckoo's Nest*. Behind this metaphor lies the philosophical conceit that the presumably insane are, in fact, saner than the normal inhabitants of a mad world. It recalls the twelfth-century Merlin who was called mad because he refused to return to the society of the Britons, whom he called the "mad, raging Britons," with their wars and their gluttony for material comforts. The moral lesson here is that all those innocent of the corruptions of the prosperous, practical pursuits of the world are called mad, but they are God's reasonable men, the poor in spirit who will inherit the kingdom of heaven. This conceit blooms most brilliantly in the Renaissance praises of folly and continues to flourish in the nineteenth century in Dostoevsky's *The Idiot* and in subtler psychiatric forms in the twentieth century. R. D. Laing's theory is that the insane often have a greater clarity and logic than the sane. The opposite side of the same coin is the metaphor of the ship of fools, according to which the world is a ship freighted with the idiocies of evil men. It found its most famous medieval spokesman in Sebastian Brant and its modern American spokesman in Katherine Anne Porter.

Behind these metaphors of a chaotic world lies the more immediate fear that not only the rest of the world but each of us is going mad. "Am I going crazy?" is a common question which expresses the terror of the loss of the self. Instead of fearing, like the medieval man, that we are falling into sin and losing our souls, we who live in the intellectual world of physiological and psychological orientation fear that we may "lose our minds." If the medieval man was most terrified that he would lose his immortal part, the soul, we fear most that we will lose what makes us mortal, our rational powers. Yet it was in the Middle Ages that men first began the long progress toward the predominance of interiorization. The devil was a powerful force who caused his worst mischief by entering *into* a man, yet man increasingly held himself responsible for submitting his will to the temptations of evil and over-indulgence which caused imbalance of the mind. If he were penitent, he could go to a priest to confess his sins and with the performance of an assigned penance he could be absolved of the sin so fully that he could enter the kingdom of paradise. Today, the problem is not so easily solved by the ordinary man. He has come to believe that the real devils of insanity lie entirely within his own mind and that he alone must expel them. For some time now, we have lived in a guilt culture, a culture which is controlled by our judgments of ourselves, rather than a shame culture, one in which our actions are controlled not by conscience, the inner voice, but by the criticism, discipline and chastisement of our peers or elders.[25] In our culture, the child is, psychiatrically speaking, the audience of the parents' moral dicta. As he grows up, however, he is supposed to interiorize this voice so that he becomes his own authority. In "A Country Doctor," Kafka's physician complains that the people want the physician to assume the role the priest once played, to take upon himself the scourges of illness. Presumably, the psychiatrist must play that role for the mental patient. The difference, unfortunately, is that, although the psychiatrist may, like the priest, offer absolution, he knows that the patient must accept it. It will not merely descend upon him.

Within the decade of the seventies, America with the rest of the world has turned increasingly toward the cult of the experts, toward an increasing interest in physical causes of mental illness, toward even a seemingly unrelated interest in astrology and demonology and magnetic force fields. Perhaps these phenomena are not unrelated but indicate the rejection the Greeks once experienced and the Romans experienced—the rejection of too much responsibility. The legacy of the Middle Ages was the increasing interiorization of the self and a concomitant increase in responsibility for human action. These ideas were consummated in the twentieth-century belief that we are responsible not only for our own actions but also for our own guilts, fears and obsessions. The fantasy of the 1970's has been a wish to return to an age of exorcism. We have even wished upon ourselves a nonexistent Middle Ages, one in which all mental illness could be exorcised. In that sense we look with favor upon demonic possession as a universal cause of all mental illness, for the devil has a separate existence as an external force and the path of virtue will lead us away from that devil and the abyss of insanity. This is only one aspect of medieval belief in the causes of insanity and we oversimplify it, but our simplification permits us to lay down an intolerable burden of responsibility and of mystery.

In one last sense, we are akin to the misunderstood medieval man. If R. D. Laing, among others, can teach us that the schizophrenic's world is as real as ours, but that his realities are different from ours, we should be able to perceive that, despite transchronological similarities of human nature and needs, the medieval world was also different from ours. Modern historians of psychiatry note that certain psychoses are both culture- and era-oriented. Schizophrenia in its catatonic form is more common in Europe, but has nearly disappeared in the United States. Africa has a higher incidence of hebephrenic schizophrenia. "Religious delusions are noted most frequently among Christians, less frequently among Buddhists, and least frequently among Hindus."[26] Ideas of grandeur and delusions about the end of the world also occur more frequently in the rural population, particularly among schizophrenics belonging to the Christian faith.

We enjoy laughter at some medieval beliefs and even some of the delusions of the medieval insane. But time and changes have caused a sort of cultural schizophrenia. We have forgotten that medieval reality was actually different from our reality. Where medieval perceptions differ from ours, we must realize that the elaborate host of demons and the forces of psychic pneuma had as real an existence in the Middle Ages as electrical impulses have in ours. A historical consideration must someday reveal to us the real and the ideal worlds against which we measure the false or true, the normal or abnormal working of the human mind.

# NOTES

## Introduction

1. Milton Rokeach, *The Three Christs of Ypsilanti* (New York: Alfred A. Knopf, 1964).

## Chapter I

1. R. G. Collingwood, *The Idea of History* (1946; New York: Oxford University Press, 1956), p. 231.

2. Constantius Africanus, *Liber de Oblivione*, in Isaac Judaeus, *Opera Omnia* (Leyden: Bartholomeus Trot, 1515), fols. ccix–cx, my translation from the Latin. Where Latin texts have been used, the translations are my own, except in large portions of Chapter III. All further citations from Constantius are from this edition and will be indicated as Constantius.

3. Galen, *On the Usefulness of the Parts of the Human Body*, ed. and trans. Margaret Tallmadge May (2 vols.; Ithaca, N.Y.: Cornell University Press, 1968).

4. Bartholomew de Glanville, *Medical Lore*, ed. and trans. Robert Steele (London: Elliot Stock, 1893), pp. 27, 28.

5. For materials on the curriculum and development of the medical school at Salerno, see Dr. A. G. Chevalier, "The Beginnings of the School of Salerno," *CIBA Symposia*, V (1944), 1719–24.

6. Isidore of Seville, "Isidore of Seville, the Medical Writings," ed. and trans. William D. Sharpe, *Transactions of the American Philosophical Society*, New Series, LIV, No. 2 (Philadelphia, 1964), 56 ff., hereafter cited as *Isidore*.

7. *Isidore*, pp. 56, 57, 58.

8. William D. Sharpe, in *Isidore*, p. 33.

9. *Liber Tertius de Egritudinibus Chronicis, Scilicet de Mania et Melancholia, et Epilepsia, et Egritudinibus Oculorum, et Dolore Aurium et Dentium, Etc.*, in *Collectio Salernitana*, ed. Salvatore de Renzii (Naples: Tipographica del Filiatre-Sebezio, 1854), II, 658, hereafter cited as *Collectio Salernitana.*

10. Aretaeus, *On the Causes and Symptoms of Chronic Diseases, The Extant Works of Aretaeus, the Cappadocian*, ed. and trans. Francis Adams (London: Werthheimer and Co., 1856), p. 299, hereafter cited as *Aretaeus.*

11. Bartholomew Anglicus, in James J. Walsh, "Bartholomew Anglicus, *De Proprietatibus Rerum*, Seventh Book—On Medicine," *Medical Life*, XL (1933), 480.

12. Arnoldus de Villanova, *De Parte Operative*, in *Opera Omnia*, ed. Nicolai Taurelli (Basel: Conrad Waldkirch, 1585), 271 A, hereafter cited as Arnold.

13. *Collectio Salernitana*, II, 659, 660.

14. This passage is quoted from Paulus Aegineta, *The Seven Books of Paulus Aegineta*, ed. and trans. Francis Adams (London: C. and J. Adlard, 1844), I, 389, hereafter cited as Paul of Aegina. A number of medieval Arab physicians, including Haly, or Ibn, Abbas and Rhazes, give substantially the same account of the disease.

15. Bernardus de Gordonio, *Omnium Aegritudinem a Vertice ad Calcem, Opus Praeclarissimus quod Lilium Medicinae Appelatur* (Paris: Dionysius Ianotus, 1542), *De Mania et Melancholia*, cap. IX, fol. 108, hereafter cited as Bernard of Gordon.

16. Paul of Aegina, I, 391.

17. Arnold, fol. 271 A.

18. Paul of Aegina, I, 391.

19. Arnold, fol. 271 A.

20. *L'Ecole de Salèrne*, ed. and trans. Charles Daremberg and C. H. Meaux (Paris: Librairie J. B. Ballière et Fils, 1880), I, 177, 178, my translation, hereafter cited as *L'Ecole de Salèrne.*

21. *L'Ecole de Salèrne*, I, 174.

22. Sancta Hildegarda, *Causae et Curae*, ed. P. Kaiser (Leipzig: B. Teubner, 1903), pp. 143, 144.


*Chapter II*

1. Caesarius of Heisterbach, *The Dialogue on Miracles*, eds. G. G. Coulton and Eileen Power, trans. H. von E. Scott and C. C. Swinton Bland (New York: Routledge, 1929), II, 179.

2. This passage is a translation of portions of the *Rituale Romanum*, quoted in Latin in T. K. Oesterreich, *Possession: Demoniacal and Other, among Primitive Races in Antiquity, the Middle Ages, and Modern Times* (1921; New York: Richard R. Smith, 1930), pp. 103, 104.

3. Jacobus de Voragine, *The Golden Legend*, eds. and trans. Granger Ryan and Helmut Ripperger (New York: Longmans and Green, 1941; New York: Arno Press, 1969), pp. 499, 671.

4. For references to these studies, see E. R. Dodds, *The Greeks and the Irrational* (1951; Berkeley: University of California Press, 1971), Ch. III, nn. 10, 11, 12, 13, 14, 15, 16.

5. See books by Oesterreich and Dodds, and Jean LHermitte, *True and False Possession*, trans. P. J. Hepburne-Scott (New York: Hawthorn Books, 1963).

6. LHermitte, pp. 1, 14, 24.

7. Tertullian, *De Anima*, in Migne, *Patrologiae Latinae, cursus completus*, II. The translation used here is from George Boas, *Primitivism and Related Ideas in the Middle Ages* (New York: Octagon Books, 1966), p. 19.

8. St. Augustine, *On Free Will*, in *Philosophy in the Middle Ages*, eds. and trans. Arthur Hyman and James J. Walsh (New York: Harper & Row, 1967), p. 37.

9. In all cases, the translation of the Bible is the Douay-Confraternity version, in which see here Colossians 2:9, 10.

10. Plato, *Phaedo*, in the *Dialogues of Plato*, trans.

B. Jowett (2 vols.; New York, Random House, 1937), I, 464.

11. *The Last Peterborough Chronicler,* in *Middle English Literature,* eds. Charles W. Dunn and Edward T. Byrnes (New York: Harcourt Brace Jovanovich, 1973), pp. 39, 40.

12. Philip Ziegler, *The Black Death* (1969; New York: Harper & Row, 1971), p. 180. On disease and morality, see Saul N. Brody, *The Disease of the Soul: Leprosy in Medieval Literature* (Ithaca, N.Y.: Cornell University Press, 1974).

13. For a lengthier study of the tradition of Nebuchadnezzar, see Penelope B. R. Doob, *Nebuchadnezzar's Children: Conventions of Madness in Middle English Literature* (New Haven: Yale University Press, 1974). On the figure of the wild man and its tradition, see Richard Bernheimer, *Wild Men in the Middle Ages* (Cambridge: Harvard University Press, 1952).

14. Isidore of Seville, *Allegoriae quaedam scripturae sacrae,* in Migne, *Patrologia Latinae* (hereafter cited as MPL), LXXIII, 116.

15. Petrus Berchorius, *Dictionarium Morale,* in *Opera Omnia* (Antwerp: Ioannus Keerbergius, 1609), III, 722.

16. St. Maximius, *Homilia,* MPL, LVIII, 257.

17. *De Anima,* MPL, I, 683.

18. Bartholomew Anglicus, *Batman uppon Bartholome, His Book De Proprietatibus Rerum, of the Braine* (London: Thomas East, 1582), III, fol. 37.

19. See Charles A. Kerin, *The Privation of Christian Burial: An Historical Synopsis and Commentary,* The Catholic University of America Canon Law Studies, no. 136 (Washington, D.C.: Catholic University of America Press, 1941), p. 205. "There is ordinarily little danger of scandal in the granting of Christian burial to a suicide since most people at present consider suicide itself a sign of mental disorder."

20. Vincent of Beauvais, *Speculum Doctrinale, Speculum Maius,* II (Graz, Austria: Akademische Druck und Verlagsanstalt [photocopy of 1624 Douay edition], 1965), Liber IV, Cap. CXVIII, col. 367. On fools and the history of folly in the Middle Ages, see John Doran, *The History of Court Fools* (London: R. Bentley, 1858); Walter P. Kaiser, *Praisers of Folly* (Cambridge: Harvard University Press, 1963); Barbara Swain, *Fools and Folly during the Middle Ages and the Renaissance* (New York: Columbia University Press, 1932); and Enid Welsford, *The Fool* (London: Faber and Faber, 1935; New York: Anchor Books, 1961).

21. "Intellectus" is the word used in the Jerome Vulgate.

22. John of Salisbury, *Policraticus* (London: Franciscus Raphelenguius, 1595), Biber VII, Cap. XV.

23. Petrus Chrysologus, "Sermo" CXXIV, in *MPL,* CXXIX, 2001.

24. *The Lives of the Women Saints of Our Countrie of England. Also Some Other Lives of Holie Women Written by Some of The Auncient Fathers* (c. 1610–15) ed. C. Horstman, Early English Text Society, Old Series 86 (London: N. Trübner, 1886), pp. 127, 128. These particular passages are actually taken from a saint's life called "The Life of St. Monica Widow, written by St. Augustine Her Sonne."

25. LHermitte, p. 115.

26. Oesterreich, p. 389.

## Chapter III

1. Reverend William M. Van Ommeren, *Mental Illness Affecting Matrimonial Consent,* The Catholic University of America Canon Law Studies, no. 415 (Washington, D.C.: Catholic University of America Press, 1961), p. 22.

2. Reverend Gennaro J. Sesto, *Guardians of the Mentally Ill in Ecclesiastical Trials,* The Catholic University of

America Canon Law Studies, no. 358 (Washington, D.C.: Catholic University of America Press, 1956), p. 21.

3. H. F. Jolowicz, *Historical Introduction to the Study of Roman Law* (1932; Cambridge: Cambridge University Press, 1967), pp. 6, 489–597.

4. A number of canonists maintain that the lawyers could not consult medical criteria for insanity because they were not available. Reference to Chapter I, on medicine, demonstrates that medical criteria were ample and available.

5. For all quotations from Roman law, except those available in the canon law studies from the Catholic University of America, I have used the translation of the *Corpus iuris civilis* and the Twelve Tables, the *Institutes of Gaius*, the *Opinions of Paulus*, which appear in the translation by S. P. Scott, *The Civil Law*, 17 vols. in 7 vols. (Cincinnati: Central Trust Company, 1932). Since Scott's references can be most easily followed by reference to his volume and page number and his item number on the page, I shall refer to the law cited by the Justinian Roman law Book and Title, but will substitute the item number and page and volume number peculiar to Scott's translation, rather than to Justinian's system. The first reference is Law Seven from the Twelve Tables, Scott, I, 67.

6. This translation from the *Institutes of Gaius* appears in Reverend Colin R. Pickett, *Mental Affliction and Church Law* (Ottawa: University of Ottawa Press, 1952), p. 13.

7. Jolowicz, pp. 130 ff.

8. Pickett, p. 22.

9. C. (5.70), 3; Scott, XIII, 276.

10. D. (27.10), 7; Scott, VI, 176.

11. D. (27.10), 11; Scott VI, 177.

12. D. (I.17), 14; Scott, II, 259.

13. *Opinions of Paulus* (IV.2); Scott, I, 312.

14. C. (5.70), 6; Scott, XIII, 277.

15. D. (24.3), 7; Scott, VI, 11.

16. D. (24.3), 7, 9, 10; Scott, VI, 11, 12.

17. D. (24.3), 7–9; Scott, VI, 11, 12.

18. D. (24.3), 8; Scott, VI, 12.

19. Ibid.

20. D. (24.3), 7; ibid.

21. For the section of waiting periods, I am indebted to Pickett, pp. 16, 17.

22. C. (1.4), 21; Scott, XII, 62.

23. D. (27.10), 11; Scott, VI, 177.

24. D. (27.10), 12; Scott, VI, 177–78.

25. D. (5.70), 5; Scott, XIII, 279.

26. C. (1.4), 21; Scott, XII, 62.

27. D. (27.10), 6; Scott, VI, 176.

28. C. (5.70), 6; Scott, XIII, 279.

29. D. (1.5), 20; Scott, II, 230.

30. D. (50.17), 124; Scott, XI, 309.

31. St. Augustine, *The City of God,* trans. Marcus Dods (New York: Modern Library, 1950), pp. 238 ff.

32. Pickett, p. 51.

33. All citations from the *Corpus iuris canonici* are from the 1959 reprint of Aemilius Richter's edition of the 1879–81 Friedberg edition of Leipzig (2 vols.; Graz, Austria: Akademische Druck und Verlagsanstalt, 1959). The standard form of notation will be used. This portion appears in C.3, C.XV, q.1.

34. On the administration of the sacraments, especially baptism, see Pickett, pp. 29 ff. On the copula theory, see Van Ommeren, pp. 13–21.

35. C.5, C.XXXIII.

36. Ibid.

37. C.14, C.XV, q.1.

38. C.12, C.XV, q.1.

39. C.3, D.XXXIII.

40. See Pickett, p. 9, and C.3, D.XXXIII.

41. C.1, C.XV, q.1.

42. Ibid.

43. C.5, C.XV, q.1.

44. C.10, C.XV, q.1.

45. C.2, C.XV, q.1.

46. C.10, C.XV, q.1.

47. C.2, C.XV, q.1.

48. C.9, C.XV, q.1.

49. C.3, D.VI.

50. C.1, D.VI.

51. C.6, C.XV, q.1.

52. C.2, C.XV, q.1.

53. Ibid.

54. C.12, C.XV, q.1.

55. C.2, C.XV, q.1.

56. C.7, C.XV, q.1.

57. This edict of 362 is translated in P. R. Coleman-Norton, *Roman State and Christian Church* (2 vols.; London: S.P.C.K., 1966), and appears in I, 279.

58. *The Bigotian Penitential*, in *Medieval Handbooks of Penance*, eds. and trans. John T. McNeill and Helen M. Gamer, *Columbia University Records of Civilization* (New York: Columbia University Press, 1938), p. 166.

59. This edict of 431 appears in Coleman-Norton, II, 655.

60. Mandate of Justinian, I, 530, in Coleman-Norton, II, 1065.

61. Sesto, p. 19.

62. See Sesto, p. 67.

63. C.15, D.XXVI.

64. C.3, D.VI.

65. St. Thomas Aquinas, *Summa Theologica*, II, q.94, a.4, ad.3, in *Treatise on Law*, ed. Stanley Parry (Chicago: Henry Regnery Co., 1970), p. 67.

66. W. S. Holdsworth, *The History of English Law* (1st. ed.; London: Methuen and Co., 1903), I, 473.

67. Sir Frederick Pollack and F. W. Maitland, *The History of English Law Before the Time of Edward I* (2nd

ed.; Cambridge: Cambridge University Press, 1898), I, 481.

68. *Senchus Mor*, eds. and trans. J. O'Donovan, T. O'Mahony, W. Neilson Hancock et al. (Dublin: Alexander Thom; London: Longmans Green, Reader and Dyer, 1865–1901), III, iiii.

69. Ibid., II, xxix.

70. Ibid., II, 407.

## Chapter IV

1. For the reference to Hoccleve's madness, I am indebted to P. R. Doob.

2. The first sections of quotation from Froissart are from the original translation by Sir John Bourchier, Lord Berners (6 vols.; London: David Nutt, 1903). All of the sections quoted from Lord Berners' sixteenth-century translation appear in VI, 61–71. I have used this translation in sections which demand a clearer sense of the spirit of Froissart's work, but I have modernized some of the more difficult spellings. When the Renaissance English becomes a hindrance, I have used the later two-volume translation of Froissart by Thomas Johnes (London: William Smith, 1929).

3. From this point on the quotations are from the Johnes edition, II, 533–46.

4. Margery Kempe, *The Book of Margery Kempe*, ed. Sanford Brown Meech, Early English Text Society, CCXII (London: Oxford University Press, 1940), 2, 3.

5. Ibid., p. 138.

6. Ibid., p. 165.

7. Ibid., pp. 177, 179 ff. All of the succeeding Kempe passages are from these pages.

8. All quotations of the "biography" are from Ernst Kris, *Psychoanalytic Explorations in Art* (1952; London: George Allen and Unwin, 1953). For this section see pp. 118, 119 ff.

9. Kris pointed out this quality of schizophrenic art, which was unusual in the Middle Ages.

10. This translation and account is from Raymond Klibansky, Erwin Panofsky and Fritz Saxl, *Saturn and Melancholy: Studies in the History of Natural Philosophy, Religion and Art* (New York: Basic Books, 1964), pp. 80, 81.

11. William Langland, *Piers the Plowman and Richard the Redeless*, ed. W. W. Skeat (2 vols.; London: Oxford University Press, 1886, 1961), I, C, Passus X, 11, 106–38.

12. See Michel Foucault, *Madness and Civilization: A History of Insanity*, trans. Richard Howard (New York: New American Library, 1967), pp. 18, 19.

13. Alfred Canel, *Recherches historiques sur les fous des Rois de France* (Paris: Alphonse Lemerre, 1873), pp. 21 ff.

14. On the origins and myths of the wild men, see Richard Bernheimer, *Wild Men in the Middle Ages* (Cambridge: Harvard University Press, 1952), which discusses the storm god and pagan religions.

15. Franz G. Alexander and Sheldon T. Selesnick, *The History of Psychiatry: An Evaluation of Psychiatric Thought and Practice from Prehistoric Times to the Present* (New York: Harper & Row, 1966), p. 64.

16. Mary Rotha Clay, *Medieval Hospitals of England*, ed. J. Charles Cox (London: Methuen and Co., 1909), p. 31.

17. Ibid., p. 34.

18. Ibid., pp. 32, 33.

19. Ibid., p. 33.

20. Foucault, p. 15.

21. Ibid., pp. 67, 68.

22. On order and the extraordinary knight, see Bernard Willson, "Ordo and Inordinatio in the Nibelungenlied," *Beiträge zur Geschichte der deutschen Sprache und Literatur* (1963), pp. 83–101.

*Chapter V*

1. Heinz E. Lehman, "Schizophrenia. IV: Clinical Features," in *Comprehensive Textbook of Psychiatry*, eds. Alfred M. Freedman and Harold I. Kaplan (Baltimore: The Williams and Wilkins Company, 1967), p. 621. The later summary of Bleuler is also Lehman's.

2. Abraham S. Goldstein, *The Insanity Defense* (New Haven: Yale University Press, 1967), quoted in Herbert Fingarette, *The Meaning of Criminal Insanity* (Berkeley: University of California Press, 1972), p. 1.

3. Henry Brill, "Classification in Psychiatry, Nosology," in Freedman and Kaplan, p. 584.

4. Milton H. Miller, "Neurosis, Psychosis, and the Borderline States," in Freedman and Kaplan, p. 590.

5. Ibid.

6. See Chapter I for the sources of all classical, Byzantine and medieval materials quoted in this chapter.

7. This statement appears in the *Collectio Salernitana*, II, 659, 660.

8. Robert A. Cohen, "Psychotic Disorders. III: Affective Reactions," in Freedman and Kaplan, p. 676.

9. See his remarks in "Psychotic Depressive Reaction," in Freedman and Kaplan, pp. 688 ff.

10. Robert A. Cohen, in Freedman and Kaplan, pp. 678, 679.

11. Milton Greenblatt, "Psychosurgery," in Freedman and Kaplan, p. 1291.

12. *Laws Governing the Hospitalization of the Mentally Ill*, VI (May 1966), 156.

13. Bruce Ennis and Loren Siegel, *The Rights of Mental Patients: The Basic ACLU Guide to a Mental Patient's Rights* (New York: Avon Books, 1973), p. 11.

14. This quotation of the law is from Fingarette, pp. 11, 12.

15. Ibid., p. 13.

16. Ibid., p. 11.

17. *Laws Governing the Hospitalization of the Mentally Ill*, p. 156.

18. § 1-05-17.

19. Philip Q. Roche's statement, from a paper published in 1958, appears in Fingarette, p. 26, n. 12.

20. § 2-74.

21. The New York State Mental Hygiene Law of 1973 makes clear and specific provisions for the conditions under which the director of a mental hospital may, at his discretion, sell the personal effects of a patient "incapable of making a rational decision," in order to pay for the patient's maintenance.

22. The information on state provisions is from Ennis and Siegel's summary of pocket versions of state mental-hygiene laws.

23. This information is also from Ennis and Siegel's summary.

24. See the definitive psychiatric article written by Victor Tausk in 1919, "On the Origin of the 'Influencing Machine' in Schizophrenia," in the *Psychoanalytic Reader* I (1948), 52–85.

25. For a brilliant early discussion of the shame and guilt cultures, see E. R. Dodds, *The Greeks and the Irrational* (1951; Berkeley: University of California Press, 1971).

26. Heinz E. Lehman, in Freedman and Kaplan, p. 641.

# BIBLIOGRAPHY

Alexander, Franz G., and Selesnick, Sheldon T. *The History of Psychiatry: An Evaluation of Psychiatric Thought and Practice from Prehistoric Times to the Present*. New York: Harper & Row, 1966.

Aretaeus. *On the Causes and Symptoms of Chronic Diseases, The Extant Works of Aretaeus, the Cappadocian*, ed. and trans. Francis Adams. London: Werthheimer and Co., 1856.

Arnoldus de Villanova. *Opera Omnia*, ed. Nicolai Taurelli. Basel: Conrad Waldkirch, 1585.

Augustine, St. *On Free Will*. In *Philosophy in the Middle Ages*, eds. and trans. Arthur Hyman and James J. Walsh. New York: Harper & Row, 1967.

——. *The City of God*, trans. Marcus Dods. New York: Modern Library, 1950.

Aurelianus, Caelius. *On Acute Disease and On Chronic Disease*, ed. I. E. Drabkin. Chicago: University of Chicago Press, 1950.

Aurelius, St. "Sermo de Calendiis Januarius," "Sermo CXXIV." In Migne, *Patrologiae Latinae*, XXXIX.

Avicenna. *Avicenna's Psychology*, trans. F. Rahman. Oxford: Oxford University Press, 1952.

Bartholomew Anglicus. *Batman uppon Bartholome, His Book De Proprietatibus Rerum*. London: Thomas East, 1582.

——. In James J. Walsh, "*De Proprietatibus Rerum*, Seventh Book—On Medicine," *Medical Life*, XL (1933), 453–96.

—— (de Glanville). *Medical Lore*, ed. and trans. Robert Steele. London: Elliot Stock, 1893.

Berchorius, Petrus. *Opera Omnia*. 3 vols. Antwerp: Ioannus Keerbergius, 1609.

Bernardus de Gordonio. *Omnium Aegritudinem a Vertice ad Calcem, Opus Praeclarissimus quod Lilium Medicinae Appelatur.* Paris: Dionysius Ianotus, 1542.

Bernheimer, Richard. *Wild Men in the Middle Ages.* Cambridge: Harvard University Press, 1952.

Blatty, William Peter. *The Exorcist.* New York: Harper & Row, 1971.

Bible. *Biblia Sacra,* eds. the monks of St. Benedict under the auspices of Pope Pius XI. 12 vols. Rome: The Vatican Press, 1926–64.

Bracton, Henricus de. *De Legibus et Consuetudinibus Angliae,* ed. Sir Travers Twiss. 6 vols. London: Longman and Co., 1878–83.

Brill, Henry D., M.D. "Nosology." In Freedman and Kaplan, eds., pp. 581–89.

Brody, Saul N. *The Disease of the Soul: Leprosy in Medieval Literature.* Ithaca: Cornell University Press, 1974.

Caesarius of Heisterbach. *The Dialogue on Miracles,* eds. G. G. Coulton and Eileen Power; trans. H. von E. Scott and C. C. Swinton Bland. 2 vols. London: Routledge, 1929.

Canel, Alfred. *Recherches historiques sur les fous des Rois de France.* Paris: Alphonse Lemerre, 1873.

Chaucer, Geoffrey. *The Works of Geoffrey Chaucer* (1933), ed. F. N. Robinson. 2nd ed.; Boston: Houghton Mifflin Company, 1937.

Chevalier, Dr. A. G. "The Beginnings of the School of Salerno," *CIBA Symposia,* V (1944), 1719–24.

———. "Constantius Africanus and the Influence of the Arabs on Salerno," *CIBA Symposia,* V (1944), 1725–31.

———. "The Salernitan Physician," *CIBA Symposia,* V (1944), 1738–42.

——— and Gerlitt, John. "Famous Medical Teachers at Montpellier," *CIBA Symposia,* V (1944), 412–17.

Chrétien de Troyes, *Arthurian Romances,* trans. W. W. Comfort. London: J. M. Dent and Sons, 1914.

——. *Yvain*, ed. Mario Roques. Paris: Librairie Ancienne Honoré Champion, 1960.

Clay, Mary Rotha. *Medieval Hospitals of England*, ed. J. Charles Cox. London: Methuen and Co., 1909.

Cohen, Robert A., M.D. "Manic Depressive-Reactions." In Freedman and Kaplan, eds., pp. 676–78.

Coleman-Norton, P. R. *Roman State and Christian Church*. 2 vols. London: S.P.C.K., 1966.

*Collectio Salernitana*, ed. Salvatore de Renzii. 5 vols. Naples: Tipografica del Filiatre-Sebezio, 1854.

Collingwood, R. G. *The Idea of History* (1946). New York: Oxford University Press, 1956.

Constantius Africanus. *Liber de Oblivione*. In Isaac Judaeus, *Opera Omnia*. Leyden: Bartholomeus Trot, 1515.

*Corpus iuris canonici*, ed. Aemilius Richter. 2 vols. Graz, Austria: Akademische Druck und Verlagsanstalt, 1959.

Dodds, E. R. *The Greeks and the Irrational* (1951). Berkeley: University of California Press, 1971.

Doob, Penelope Billings Reed. *Ego Nabugodonosor: A Study of Conventions of Madness in Middle English Literature*. Ph.D. dissertation, Stanford University, 1969.

——. *Nebuchadnezzar's Children: Conventions of Madness in Middle English Literature*. New Haven: Yale University Press, 1974.

Doran, John. *The History of Court Fools*. London: R. Bentley, 1858.

*L'Ecole de Salèrne*, ed. and trans. Charles Daremberg and C. H. Meaux. 2 vols. Paris: J.-B. Baillière et Fils, 1880.

Ennis, Bruce, and Siegel, Loren. *The Rights of Mental Patients: The Basic ACLU Guide to A Mental Patient's Rights*. New York: Avon Books, 1973.

Fingarette, Herbert. *The Meaning of Criminal Insanity* (1972). Berkeley: University of California Press, 1974.

Foucault, Michel. *Madness and Civilization: A History of Insanity*, trans. Richard Howard. New York: New American Library, 1967.

Freedman, Alfred M., and Kaplan, Harold I., eds. *Com-*

*prehensive Textbook of Psychiatry.* Baltimore: The Williams and Wilkins Company, 1967.

Froissart, Syr John. *The Cronycle of Syr John Froissart,* trans. Syr John Bourchier, Lord Berners. 6 vols. London: David Nutt, 1903.

———. *Sir John Froissart's Chronicles of England, France, Spain, & etc., & etc.,* trans. Thomas Johnes. 2 vols. London: William Smith, 1929.

Galen. *On the Usefulness of the Parts of the Human Body,* ed. and trans., Margaret Tallmadge May. 2 vols. Ithaca: Cornell University Press, 1968.

Geoffrey of Monmouth. *Vita Merlini,* ed. and trans., J. J. Parry. Illinois University Studies in Language and Literature, X (1925), 9–81.

*Gesta Romanorum,* ed. Sidney J. H. Herrtage. Early English Text Society, XXXIII. London: J. Trübner, 1879.

Green, Hannah. *I Never Promised You a Rose Garden.* New York: New American Library, 1964.

Greenblatt, Milton. "Psychosurgery." In Freedman and Kaplan, eds., pp. 1291–95.

Group for the Advancement of Psychiatry. *Laws Governing the Hospitalization of the Mentally Ill,* VI (May 1966).

Haly Abbas. *Liber totius medicine necessaria,* ed. Michaele de Capella; trans. Stephan of Antioch. Leyden: Jacob Myt, 1523.

Hildegarda, Sancta. *Causae et Curae,* ed. P. Kaiser. Leipzig: B. Teubner, 1903.

Hippocrates. *The Genuine Works of Hippocrates,* trans. Francis Adams. 2 vols. New York: William Wood and Co., 1886.

Hoccleve, Thomas. *Hoccleve's Works, The Minor Poems,* eds. Frederick J. Furnivall and I. Gollancz. Early English Text Society, E.S., 61, 73. London: Oxford University Press, 1970.

Holdsworth, W. S. *The History of English Law.* 1st ed., 16 vols. London: Methuen and Co., 1903–66.

Huston, Paul E., M.D. "Psychotic Depressive Reaction." In Freedman and Kaplan, eds., pp. 688–97.

Isidore of Seville, St. *Allegoriae quaedam scripturae sacrae*. In Migne, *Patrologiae Latinae*, LXXXIII.

——. "Isidore of Seville, the Medical Writings, Translation of Books XI and IV of the Etymologies," ed. and trans. William D. Sharpe. *Transactions of the American Philosophical Society*, New Series, Vol. LIV, No. 2. Philadelphia, 1964.

Jacobus de Voragine. *The Golden Legend*, eds. and trans. Granger Ryan and Helmut Ripperger. New York: Arno Press, 1969.

Janson, Horst W. *Apes and Ape Lore in the Middle Ages and the Renaissance*. London: The Warburg Institute, 1952.

John of Salisbury. *Policraticus*. London: Franciscus Raphelenguius, 1595.

Jolowicz, H. F. *Historical Introduction to the Study of Roman Law* (1932). Cambridge: Cambridge University Press, 1967.

Kaiser, Walter P. *Praisers of Folly*. Cambridge: Harvard University Press, 1963.

Kempe, Margery. *The Book of Margery Kempe*, ed., Sanford Brown Meech. Early English Text Society, CCXII. London: Oxford University Press, 1940.

Kerin, Charles A. *The Privation of Christian Burial: An Historical Synopsis and Commentary*. The Catholic University of America Canon Law Studies, no. 136. Washington, D.C.: Catholic University of America Press, 1941.

Kesey, Ken. *One Flew over the Cuckoo's Nest*. New York: Viking Press, 1964.

Klibansky, Raymond; Panofsky, Irwin; and Saxl, Fritz. *Saturn and Melancholy: Studies in the History of Natural Philosophy, Religion and Art*. New York: Basic Books, 1964.

Kris, Ernst. *Psychoanalytic Explorations in Art* (1952). London: George Allen and Unwin, 1953.

Kuttner, Stephan. *Kanonistische Schuldlehre von Gratian bis auf die Dekretalen Gregors IX. Studi e Testi,* 64. Vatican City, 1935.

Ladner, Gerhart B. "Homo Viator: Medieval Ideas on Alienation and Order," *Speculum,* LXII (April 1967), 233–59.

Laing, R. D. *The Divided Self: An Existential Study in Sanity and Madness.* London: Pelican Books, 1965.

Langland, William. *Piers the Plowman and Richard the Redeless* (1866), ed. W. W. Skeat. 2 vols. London: Oxford University Press, 1886, 1961.

Lehman, Heinz E., M.D. "Schizophrenia. I: Introduction and History." In Freedman and Kaplan, eds., pp. 593–99.

LHermitte, Jean. *True and False Possession,* trans. P. J. Hepburne-Scott. New York: Hawthorn Books, 1963.

*The Lives of the Women Saints of Our Countrie of England,* ed. C. Horstman. Early English Text Society, Old Series, 86. London: N. Trübner, 1886.

Mâle, Emile. *L'Art Religieux du XIIe Siècle en France.* Paris: Librairie Armand Colin, 1953.

Maximius, St. *Homilia,* XVI. In Migne, *Patrologie Latinae,* LVII.

*McKinney's Consolidated Laws of New York, Annotated Domestic Relations Law.* L. 1964, Book 14.

——. *Mental Hygiene Law.* L. 1972, c. 51 (Pocket Version), Book 34 A.

*Medieval Handbooks of Penance,* eds. and trans. John T. McNeill and Helen M. Gamer. *Columbia University Records of Civilization.* New York: Columbia University Press, 1938.

*Middle English Literature,* eds. Charles W. Dunn and Edward T. Byrnes. New York: Harcourt Brace Jovanovich, 1973.

Migne, J. P. ed., *Patrologiae cursus completus: Patrologia Latina,* 221 vols., Paris: Garnier Fratres, 1844–64.

Miller, Milton H., M.D. "Neurosis, Psychosis, and the Borderline States." In Freedman and Kaplan, eds., pp. 589–93.

O'Brien-Moore, Ainsworth. *Madness in Ancient Literature.* Ph.D. dissertation, Princeton University. Weimar: R. Wagner, 1924.

Oesterreich, T. K. *Possession: Demoniacal and Other.* New York: Richard R. Smith, 1930.

Paulus Aegineta. *The Seven Books of Paulus Aegineta,* ed. and trans. Francis Adams. 2 vols. London: C. and J. Adlard, 1844.

Petrus Chrysologus, St. "Sermo" CVL. In Migne, *Patrologiae Latinae,* LII.

Pickett, Rev. R. Colin. *Mental Affliction and Church Law.* Ph.D. dissertation, Catholic University of Ottawa. Ottawa: University of Ottawa Press, 1952.

Plato. *The Dialogues of Plato,* trans. B. Jowett. 2 vols. New York: Random House, 1937.

Pollack, Sir Frederick, and Maitland, F. W. *The History of English Law Before the Time of Edward I.* 2nd ed., 2 vols. Cambridge: Cambridge University Press, 1898.

Rokeach, Milton. *The Three Christs of Ypsilanti.* New York: Alfred A. Knopf, 1964.

*Senchus Mor.,* eds. and trans. J. O'Donovan, T. O'Mahony, W. Neilson et al. 6 vols. Dublin: Alexander Thom; London: Longmans Green, Reader and Dyer, 1865–1901.

Sesto, Rev. Gennaro J. *Guardians of the Mentally Ill in Ecclesiastical Trials.* The Catholic University of America Canon Law Studies, no. 358. Washington, D.C.: Catholic University of America Press, 1956.

Siegel, Rudolph. *Galen's System of Physiology and Medicine.* Basel and New York: S. Karger, 1968.

Simon, Bennet, and Weiner, Herbert. "Models of Mind and Mental Illness in Ancient Greece: I. The Homeric

Mind," *Journal of the History of the Behavioral Sciences,* II (1966), 303–14.

Singer, Samuel. *Sprichwörter des Mittelalters.* 3 vols. Bern: Herbert Lang et Cie., 1944–47.

Swain, Barbara. *Fools and Folly during the Middle Ages and the Renaissance.* New York: Columbia University Press, 1932.

Tausk, Victor. "On the Origin of the 'Influencing Machine' in Schizophrenia" (1933). *Psychoanalytical Reader,* I (1948), 52–85.

Tertullian. *De Anima.* In Migne, *Patrologiae Latinae,* II.

Thomas Aquinas, St. *Treatise on Law,* ed. Stanley Parry. Chicago: Henry Regnery Co., 1970.

Thorndike, Lynn. *The History of Magic and Experimental Science.* 7 vols. New York: The Macmillan Company and Columbia University Press, 1923–58.

Van Ommeren, Rev. William M. *Mental Illness Affecting Matrimonial Consent.* The Catholic University of America Canon Law Studies, no. 415. Washington, D.C.: Catholic University of America Press, 1961.

Vaughan, Agnes Carr. *Madness in Greek Thought and Custom.* Baltimore: J. H. Furst and Company, 1919.

Vincent of Beauvais. *Speculum Doctrinale, Speculum Maius,* II. Graz, Austria: Akademische Druck und Verlagsanstalt (photocopy of 1624 Douay edition), 1965.

Welsford, Enid. *The Fool.* London: Faber and Faber, 1935; New York: Anchor Books, 1961.

White, Lynn, Jr. *Medieval Technology and Social Change* (1962). Oxford: Oxford University Press, 1963.

Whitwell, J. R. *Historical Notes on Psychiatry.* 2 vols. London: H. K. Lewis and Co., 1936.

Willson, Bernard. "Ordo and Inordinatio in the Nibelungenlied," *Beiträge zur Geschichte der deutschen Sprache und Literatur,* CXXXV (Tübingen, 1963), 83–101.

Wolberon. *Commentaria in Cantum Canticorum.* In Migne, *Patrologiae Latinae,* CXVC.

Wolfson, Harry Austryn. *The Philosophy of the Church Fathers* (1956). Cambridge: Harvard University Press, 1970.

——. *Studies in the History of Philosophy and Religion,* Vol. I, eds. Isadore Twersky and George H. Williams. Cambridge: Harvard University Press, 1973.

*Ywain and Gawain,* ed. G. Schleich. Leipzig: Eugen Franck, 1887.

Ziegler, Philip. *The Black Death* (1969). New York: Harper & Row, 1971.

Zilboorg, Gregory. *A History of Medical Psychology.* New York: W. W. Norton and Co., 1941.

# INDEX